KETO DIET ADVANCED

Keto Diet Plan to Healthy Eating and Detox for Weight Loss

By

Harry Humble

Table of Contents

Introduction 1

Chapter 1 The Trend Of Ketogenic Dieting 3

Chapter 2 Advantages Of The Ketogenic Diet 7

Chapter 3 Why Choosing Ketogenic Lifestyle 11

Chapter 4 How The Ketogenic Diet Works 14

Chapter 5 Feed Controversy 17

Chapter 6 The Healthy Low Carbohydrate Approach 20

Chapter 7 How Are Ketogenic Diets' Done Right' 23

Chapter 8 How Do You Know If You're Burning Fat? 29

Chapter 9 The Science Behind Ketosis 34

Chapter 10 The Science Behind 7 Keto DHEA 38

Chapter 11 Fat And Protein Ratio In A Ketogenic Diet 47

Chapter 12 Is The Keto Diet Plan Safe For You? 50

Chapter 13 Keto Diet And Plant Based Eating 57

Chapter 14 Analysing Your Weight Loss Objectives 62

Chapter 15 Ketogenic Diet For Treating Type 1 & 2 Diabetes ... 65

Chapter 16 Keto For Lowering Convulsions 74

Chapter 17 Aerobic Exercise And Ketogenic Weight Loss Plan .. 78

Chapter 18 Ketogenic Diet For Bipolar Patients 84

Chapter 19 Ketogenic Dieting For Treating Migraines 87

Chapter 20 Sugar, Fat And Protein Precaution On The Ketogenic Diet ... 90

Chapter 21 What Foods To Avoid On The Keto Diet? 99

Chapter 22 Changing Your Food Environment 102

Chapter 23 The Unwanted Side Effects Of Using A Ketogenic Diet
For Weight Loss 106

Chapter 24 What's The Proof That Ketogenic Diet Works? 109

Chapter 25 Rules For A Headache- Free Ketogenic Diet 114

Chapter 26 How To Beat Keto Flu 118

Chapter 27 Achieve Success With Advanced Ketogenic Diet 120

Chapter 28 Tips To Make Ketogenic Diet Work 125

Conclusion 130

Introduction

The ketogenic weight loss program is an eating plan according to a procedure known as ketosis. It is a certain status of the entire body that is recognized by an elevated level of ketones of the bloodstream, which happens because of the transformation of fat into fatty ketones and acids.

This occurs once the body gets just tiny amounts of carbohydrates over a particular time. If you begin with this diet type, the body goes through many changes. Within 24-48 hours of the start of the diet plan, the entire body starts to make use of ketones i.e. the energy kept in fat cells better.

Put simply, the main source of energy turns into body fat (fatty acids), rather than carbohydrates (glucose). Due to that, throughout ketosis, it is not really an issue to consume meals with increased quantities of excess fat than would usually appear realistic.

This particular manner, the body is fast losing weight (specifically fat). Additionally, the loss of muscle tissue (proteins) is very little, since the great bulk of foods consumed throughout ketosis, additionally has fairly a lot of proteins which are great for the muscles.

Even though ketosis is the foundation of the ketogenic diet type, in its strictest form it does not have to be maintained for very long. The state of ketosis may be held up until the weight is merely a couple of pounds higher than what is desired. Afterward, foods with higher quantities of carbs are slowly introduced (rice, beans,...).

In this particular period, it will be very helpful to keep a food consumption diary where regular amounts of taken carbs will be observed. The way you can discover the maximum amount of everyday carbs that nonetheless allows you never to gain weight.

When you learn this particular parameter, you'll not have heavy related issues, because, until that moment, you'll definitely discover how to have an account of amounts and calories of carbohydrates, fats, and proteins which you eat every day.

The approach you will get to know the body much better, in the terminology of the optimum "allowable" daily intake. Due to that, we can say the ketogenic diet plan is, a process for learning habits which will see to it that you never ever go back to the existing tricky obese amounts.

You will find numerous kinds of ketogenic diet programs which are available in different sources, though they almost all have in typical one fundamental concept - intake of high quantities of fats and proteins, and little amounts of carbs.

This **ADVANCED GUIDE** on **KETOGENIC DIET** is fully packed with facts and information to assist you in your journey on **KETO DIETING**.

Chapter 1
The Trend Of Ketogenic Dieting

Keto diet has gained popularity in recent years and has become a nutritional plan favored by all ages. That said, this dietary roadmap may precipitate particularly important health benefits for people over 50.

A scientifically classified ketogenic diet, this nutritional plan stresses reduced carbohydrate food consumption and increased fat intake. Low carbohydrate intake is said to eventually place the participating dietary bodies in a biological and metabolic process known as ketosis.

Once ketosis is established, the body becomes particularly efficient in burning fat and turning these substances into energy. Furthermore, during this process, the body is thought to metabolize fat into chemicals classified as ketones, which are also said to provide significant energy sources.

An accelerator is an intermittent fasting method that causes your body to access the next available energy source or ketones from stored fat. Without glucose, the body now burns fat for energy.

There are a number of other specific ketogenic diets, including targeted (TKD) diets that gradually add small amounts of carbohydrates to their diet.

Cyclical (CKD)

Adherents to this plan consume carbohydrates cyclically like every few days or weeks.

High-protein

High-protein dieters do eat more protein in their dietary plans.

Standard (SKD)

Typically, this most commonly used version of dietary intake significantly reduced carbohydrate concentrations (maybe as little as five percent of all dietary intake), along with protein-laden foods and high-fat products (in some cases as much as 75 percent of all dietary needs).

The average dieter or someone new to the keto diet mostly participate in standard or high-protein versions. Professional athletes or people with very specific dietary requirements usually undertake cyclical and targeted variations.

Recommended Foods Keto diet adherents are encouraged to eat foods such as meat, fatty fish, dairy products such as cheeses, milk, butter and cream, eggs, produce low-carbohydrate products, condiments such as salt, pepper and a host of other spices, various needs and seeds and oils such as olive and coconut.

However, certain foods should be avoided or strictly limited. Such items include beans and legumes, many fruits, high-sugar edibles, alcohol and grain products.

Keto diet adherents, aged 50 and above, do enjoy numerous health benefits such as Increased mental and physical energy As people grow older, energy levels may drop for a variety of environmental and biological reasons. Keto diet followers often see strength and vitality boost.

One reason the occurrence is because the body burns excess fat, which is synthesized into energy. Moreover, ketone synthesis tends to increase brain power and stimulate cognitive functions such as focus and memory.

Improved sleepers tend to sleep less as they age. Keto dieters often gain more from exercise programs and become easier tired. Such occurrence could precipitate longer, more fruitful rest periods.

Metabolism

Aging individuals often experience slower metabolism than in their younger days. Long-term keto dieters experience greater blood sugar regulation, which can increase metabolic rates.

Weight loss

Faster and more efficient fat metabolism helps eliminate accumulated body fat, which could precipitate excess pound shedding. Also, followers are believed to have a reduced appetite that could result in reduced caloric intake.

Keeping off the weight is important, especially as adults age when they may need fewer calories daily compared to living in their 20s or 30s. Yet getting nutrient-rich food from this diet for older adults still matters.

Because aging adults often lose muscle and strength, a nutritionist may recommend a high protein-specific ketogenic diet.

Protection Against Specific Illnesses

Keto dieters over the age of 50 may reduce their risk of developing ailments such as diabetes, mental disorders such as Alzheimer's, various cardiovascular diseases, various cancers, Parkinson's disease, non-alcoholic fatty liver disease (NAFLD) and multiple sclerosis.

Some consider aging the most important risk factor for human disease or disease. Reducing aging is the logical step to minimize disease risk factors.

Good news from the description of the ketosis process discussed above shows that increased energy of the youth as a result and because of the use of fat as a fuel source, the body can go through a process where signs can be misinterpreted so that the mTOR signal is suppressed and a lack of glucose is evident where aging is reported to be slowed.

Multiple studies have generally observed for years that caloric restriction can help slow aging and boost lifespan. With the ketogenic diet, it is possible to affect anti-aging without reducing calories. An intermittent fasting method used with the keto diet may also affect vascular aging.

When a person fasts intermittently or on a keto diet, it is believed that BHB or Beta-Hydroxybutyrate induces anti-aging effects.

Ketogenic diets, which are very low in carbohydrates and usually high in fats and/or proteins, are used to treat obesity and cardiovascular diseases effectively in weight loss.

An important note in the chapter, however, was that " the impact of keto diets on cardiovascular risk factors are also controversial" and likewise, these diets are not totally safe and can be associated with some adverse events."

Chapter 2
Advantages Of The Ketogenic Diet

For decades, you've heard that you're fat. Your body is constructed to use fat as an alternative fuel source. For most of history, people didn't eat three square meals and snacks all day long.

Instead, humans would have to hunt and collect their food, and they learned to flourish when no food was accessible, sometimes for days to end. They used fat for energy to keep going. Thank you, evolution.

Here are just a few advantages of a ketogenic diet filled with high-quality fats:

Burns body fat: when you are on the keto diet, your body uses stored body fat as fuel. The lead?

Quick weight loss.

Reduces appetite: ketones also suppress ghrelin— your hormone in starvation and boost CCK cholecystokinin that makes you feel complete. Reduced appetite means it's simple and easier to go without eating for longer periods, encouraging your body to use its stored fat for energy.

Reduces inflammation: Too much inflammation is bad news because it increases chronic disease risk. A keto diet can reduce inflammation in the body by producing fewer free radicals than glucose and turning off inflammatory pathways.

Fuels your brain: Ketones are so strong that they can provide up to 20 percent of your brain's energy requirements, which is much more effective than glucose energy. Did you know your brain is more than 60% fat?

It requires lots of fat to maintain the engine moaning. On a ketogenic diet, the healthy fats you consume more than feed your daily activities— they also feed your brain.

Increases power: when your brain uses fuel ketones, when you eat lots of carbs, you don't experience the same energy slumps. When your metabolism is fat-burning, your body can tap its readily accessible energy fat stores.

No more crashes or brain fog. Also ketosis enables the brain generate more mitochondria, cell power generators. More energy in your cells means more energy.

Fat is a super-satisfying macronutrient. You eat a ton of good keto fats, so you feel thicker.

You tend to avoid experiencing blood sugar swings and cravings that plague most individuals on the Standard American Diet when you begin eating more fat and cutting all additional carbs (think sugar, bread and pasta).

When your body works on fuel ketones, it constantly supplies body fat energy. When your body depends on glucose, it needs regular hit carbs to keep it going.

Ketones can control hunger and satiety hormones so you feel fulfilled, full, not hungry. That implies fewer hunger, more energy, and fat-burning. Operates here.

How ketones influence your hunger hormones Ketones influence cholecystokinin (CCK), a hormone that makes you feel complete, and ghrelin, the "hunger hormone."

CCK: your intestines release CCK after you consume, and it's a strong food intake regulator— so much so that injecting individuals with CCK will cause them to shorten their meals.[9] Ketones boost CCK concentrations so that after meals you're happy.

Ghrelin: Ghrelin is called "hunger hormone" as it enhances appetite. It's released from your stomach and intestines, with blood levels peaking at fasting.

When you lastly consume a meal, ghrelin falls to blood nutrients. Ketosis suppresses ghrelin weight-loss increase. So when you're in ketosis, you don't think about your next meal.

One reason calorie-restricted diets tend to fail is that these diets make you really hungry, causing cravings in food.

Cutting calories to lose excess weight shifts your hormones. After you're hungry enough to lose weight, your brain and gut begin working against you. Your hormones shout, "Eat more and recover that weight." A nutritional yo-yo lifetime starts.

But it's not that way. Skip the calorie-restriction, hungry-all-time thing, and make complete use of ketosis without getting hungry. As long as you consume mild protein, a larger percentage of fat, and minimal carbs, you'll feel energized and happy.

The keto diet is fairly easy: consume mostly healthy fats (75% of your daily calories), some protein (20%), and very tiny carbs (5%). This combination puts you in ketosis.

Choose products like meat, fish, eggs, vegetables, and fat. Check this comprehensive keto food list and browse these meal ideas recipes. Most individuals consume 30 to 150 grams of net carbs everyday.

"Net carbs" implies you can remove sugar alcohols like xylitol and fibre from your usual carb count— they do not affect your blood sugar or store it as glucose storage form.

Chapter 3
Why Choosing Ketogenic Lifestyle

Ketogenic diet is a low-carb diet. High-fat, mild protein, low-carb diet. It makes your body fat-burning. There's a much more science explanation, but you basically force your body to generate energy ketones in the liver. On the other hand, eating high-carbs and sugars foods your body will produce glucose and raise insulin levels.

Ketogenics, though new to many, has been around since the 1920s. Clinical Nutrition's American Journal released many studies. Studies found documented weight loss and attendees consumed less food.

To enter ketosis, decrease your carbs to below 50 grams a day. Max. Thirty-five carbs. Your fat consumption should be about 75% meal and about 15% protein. It varies from person to person, but you should get ketosis within 3-14 days.

When consuming elevated carbohydrates, your metabolism usually burns carbs for fuel. Never burn stored fat. If you reduce the carbs available, your body must burn your fat.

If you consider these dietary changes, you should always check with your doctor. Keto's changing lifestyle. You're changing how you eat. To succeed, you should be consistent and consider long-term consequences.

Initially, when I started examining ketogenic eating, my primary goal was to shed extra pounds. I'm what I call "recovering fatass," just as someone who has stopped drinking might well be known as "recovering alcoholic."

I've struggled with my weight all my life, and I fully expect that even if I can accomplish the goals I've chosen (and I'll), the fight won't be over. I think it's an important realization for anyone trying to lose weight, but that's another day's theme.

The first thing that drew me into a ketogenic diet as a way to lose weight was whenever you strictly limit your carbohydrate intake, you'll be able to force (I'm keen to say "train") your system to choose fat as fuel, as opposed to carbs. I'm interested in life-hacking and "mind over matter," and the simple fact I'd take over my body became a big incentive.

Besides the premise that I could train my body to use fat as fuel, the claims of reduced hunger and appetite attracted me. As anyone who has ever experienced diet before knows, hunger pangs are usually awful to manage, and when willpower slips at the wrong time it's not hard to get rid of a week worth careful eating with one binge.

Many people generally say that after a limited time eating a ketogenic diet (mostly 2-4 weeks), they often find that they are not as hungry as they were before, even on a calorie-reduced diet. Not being hungry means less chance of messing up on a diet plan, which is a big plus for me.

Finally, I was fascinated by the food I could eat and keep my ketogenic diet. I've been inquisitive about food beyond eating for ages, so I enjoy cooking a lot, of course, if you find one of the main truths about food, it's that fat is the flavor.

A diet program that allowed but encouraged fat as the food was like discovering the ultimate goal. However, as I told anyone I've discussed ketogenic eating with, it's not a diet plan that suggests you can eat whatever you want in whatever quantity.

Mathematically, losing weight is... If you eat less than you spend, you can expect the weight to drop, full stop. But by making the calories I take in delicious, I won't crave extras, and I'll be more likely to follow my plan. Or at least that's theory.

So you've got it. This is just a quick guide to some of the things that drew me to ketogenic eating, another day we'll touch on the specific science behind this diet. At least now you know what moved me on my fat-burning journey.

You will hear suggestions for calculating the macros to know how much to eat. I suggest you forget about the macros, you'll be too restricted, you'll lose weight a little faster, but you'll be hungry.

The basic direction I give my clients— you want to eat a lot of fat, a moderate amount of protein, and 20 grams (or less) of carbs a day.

Determine the amount of protein by this calculation: male-50 grams of protein for the first 5 feet, add 2.3 grams for each additional inch Female-45.5 grams of protein for the first 5 feet, add 2.3 grams for each additional inch.

You'll see men starting with more protein. Ladies, that's how it works.

Once you know how much protein you need, math is done. After a few days of keeping an eye on how much protein and carbs you eat, it will become second nature for you, and you won't count anything. No more daily food.

I know everyone wants a detailed plan, but one thing I love is how flexible a ketogenic diet is. I can eat this lifestyle without stress.

Choose a high-fat meat- salami, bacon, sausage, ribeye steak, dark meat chicken, eggs. Add a high-fat blue cheese salad and a green vegetable. Then-load the fat. Cook your chicken with coconut oil and make some dressing w / mostly olive oil and less vinegar. It's simple.

Chapter 4
How The Ketogenic Diet Works

When you consume a standard carbohydrate-filled American diet, your body breaks these down into glucose that can enter your bloodstream and be used as a fuel for all your body's procedures.

But if you're hungry for carbohydrates, your body can't produce enough glucose for your energy needs. At this stage, your body will turn to a workaround: it will start looking for fat that can break down into ketones.

"Ketones are basically an alternative body fuel," Poff explains. Sometimes called "ketone bodies," they are easy compounds created by fatty acid breakdown in the liver.

"If you manipulate your diet in this high-fat, low-carb scenario, you will start making these ketones and they will increase to significant blood levels." From there, ketones will further break down to make adenosine triphosphate (ATP), the chemical that energizes your body's cells just like glucose.

The main reason for keto's growing popularity today is its alleged weight loss impact, and there is some evidence that keto can help people lose weight quicker with minimal side effects on a more traditional low-fat diet.

Studies have also shown that keto is especially helpful to those struggling to lose weight owing to metabolic disorders like insulin resistance and polycystic ovary syndrome.

Side-effects and risks must also be considered, however. During the switch to ketosis, some report exhaustion, gastrointestinal distress, and other symptoms; known as "keto flu."

People that are taking insulin-controlled medications may experience a severe complication referred to as ketoacidosis if their dosages are not adjusted before switching.

Therefore, if you attempt, the best recommendation is to work with your doctor to monitor your health throughout. Including a registered dietitian who can ensure you get the vitamins, minerals, and other nutrients you need to support your health is also a good idea.

Furthermore, the ketogenic diet has drawn science attention as a possible key to stabilizing aging and associated illnesses.

But it also turns out ketones aren't just fuel. "Ketones also signal molecules, which means they can communicate with cell membrane receptors." "They can also communicate with other cell and blood molecules."

For instance, a 2015 mice research discovered that ketones can prevent the activation of certain inflammatory chemicals that become overactivated in many chronic illnesses and aging. Another 2013 mouse research found that ketones can also up-regulate our natural antioxidant defense mechanism.

In another recent study, this one from 2018, rats fed a ketogenic diet in coenzyme nicotinamide adenine dinucleotide (NAD+), an essential protein without which your cells can not function. It is known to decrease with age, contributing to human-age breakdowns cascade.

What this means is that ketosis could help slow down aging through a variety of diverse pathways: possibly by down-regulating oxidative stress and inflammation, and increasing the presence of key longevity-significant enzymes.

The theory that ketogenic diet can help slow aging and prolong health span shows some promise in animal studies, but much more study is needed to see if this would translate into ageing.

Scientists hope the ketogenic diet may be used to treat more than seizures. A range of studies are currently underway to determine the usefulness of keto in treating certain cancers and other neurological disorders such as Parkinson's, Alzheimer's, and multiple sclerosis. But all this research is in its infancy.

"Most proof indicates that there are clear advantages of ketosis for some periods of time. Animal and human nutritional effects studies, for instance, have discovered improvements in obesity and type 2 diabetes, but only for a restricted time.

Although it is uncertain how long— and sometimes with negative side impacts such as non-alcoholic fatty liver illness and insulin re Ketones are much of how we survived. They're really essential because they're the brain's only other primary energy source outside glucose.

Chapter 5
Feed Controversy

The majority of the Western Governments provide health guidelines that ask us to base our food consumption nearly universally near grain type carbs, which were previously classified as starches. We all know these most often as rice, bread, potatoes, and pasta.

These food types seem to be staples of the western diets (they are not, but that is a different story). We are usually told that consuming these superfoods will provide us complete, full and satisfied of a slow-stream of energy that is safe and healthy. Regrettably, at least for man, this does not constantly seem to be the case.

Only some grains are created equal for a beginning and this could be where grain advocates accidentally or purposely misleading. For example, virtually all-grain, especially white rice, is going to convert to sugar fast in the system and also we have actually noticed several of the disastrous consequences of excess sugar consumption.

Grains, whatever source they are from is going to cause an elevated insulin levels. For the really good amongst us, with really sensitive insulin through great genes, a combination of regular exercise of both) might be ready to thoroughly make use of small levels of grains to fuel the bodies with the times of activity that is high.

However, for the great bulk of individuals, the excess of grains can lead to nearly all of exactly the same issues as sugar usage.

A lot of low carb exponents are distrustful of medical advice to consume cereals, several citing Government subsidies of mass farming.

Eating grains is an extremely simple and cheap way of offering food, but inexpensive and very simple is seldom just like good and healthy.

Veggies!

Low carbohydrate diet programs have usually been viewed as low in vegetables as individuals intelligently trim away almost all extra carbs, effectively throwing the baby away with the unclean bathwater. On the topic of produce, you will not find a lot of dissension amongst healthcare pros of any

standpoint. These foodstuffs not just have a plethora of minerals and vitamins, but also tend to be chock full of fiber, water and a multitude of amazing cancer-fighting substances special to vegetables.

The really important aspect of vegetables is they are nutrient-dense and calorie sparse. In plain English, they include a great deal of stuff that is good in an extremely little package. You can consume practically sufficient vegetables to fill you up but still have consumed just a small portion of the energy a typical diet would confer.

Among the arguments for normal grain ingestion will be the required minerals and vitamins they contain, and the vital fiber for the digestive tract. Vegetables make grains appear to be rather redundant.

A tiny handful of vegetables that are organic will have far more minerals and vitamins than practically a day 's worth of cereals, all in a simpler for your body to digest and process program, with no danger and extra water of insulin overload.

While on a low carb diet plan, you can stuff yourself with vegetables with no dread. The main benefit of a low carb diet is insulin control which will not interfere with that.

Remember vegetables that are organic have a substantially greater vitamin and mineral content, additionally the darker green and white a vegetable the taller the quantity of helpful Chlorophyll within the place. Try eating the veggies raw and fresh and oftentimes. A normal source of mixed veggies is as nature 's most ideal multivitamin pill.

Chapter 6
The Healthy Low Carbohydrate Approach

As a number of low carb dieters have indicated that, many people were not created to reside on high carbohydrate food in the diets. As hunter-gatherers, we consisted largely on creatures which roamed wild and on fresh berries and vegetables we were can get in the local habitat.

Even though the societies might have progressed enough to allow us to develop sustained agriculture, the genes continue to be locked in a 100 thousand-year-old fight for survival. Our bodies understand the nutrients offered from scrub clean meats, fresh vegetables, and healthy fats.

They have substantial difficulty coping with the unexpected influx of extra energy and too rapidly assimilated carbohydrates in the type of sugars and grains.

To restrict the intake of grains plus sugars makes a positive and fast fairly change towards a much healthier lifestyle.

Nevertheless, it might be that in the urge to lose weight with only a small amount ache as you possibly can, the lower carbohydrate diets we select are tilted towards the proteins and fats we do not absolutely need and focus on vegetables is dismissed.

With a few small modifications, we can get a lower carbohydrate approach that not merely allows us to have a normalized fat mass and body-weight but likewise allows us to be an all-round healthier unique.

You will find 100 other points towards enhancing health but these changes make an admirable beginning.

Eat YOUR VEGGIES! (They are the great carbohydrates & will not hinder your low carbohydrate benefits)

CHOOSE LEAN EGGS and MEATS (Eggs are a terrific source of protein and grass-fed organic meat)

Go for Better Fats (Make certain you consume a regular source of Omega three fats amongst the other daily intakes. Fat that is saturated of moderation isn't the risk. Glucose is.

Avoid SUGARS And GRAINS!

Low carb is much less about maligning one specific food group and more about keeping away from all those options that the body cannot tackle in a lot. Healthy individuals and athletes might be equipped to work with restricted sugar or grains to enhance performance but the exact same fundamental rules apply elsewhere

Drink Plenty of Water

We usually argue over what groups of foods are crucial or not but one we can all agree on is drinking water. You want it and a lot of it. Forgot food, with no water you die fast.

Be skeptical OF Special LOW CARB Foods

There are a good number of good options right here, Athletes particularly will love easy-to-mix carb totally free protein-rich drinks, etc but as low carb diet programs have hit particular meal industries tough, expect a lot of products which might be lower carbohydrate options but aren't good. Never forget the low fat craze where manufacturers swapped fat that is saturated for a lot of sugar.

Mix YOUR Food Choices

Restricting cereals and sugars is a fantastic beginning but do not get caught in the trap of merely surviving on similar meat diet day in and day out. Mix your fats and proteins and vegetables offer a multitude of good options.

Enjoy the DIET!

Just since you stopped eating bread and chips with the meals does not imply you have to get weary! There is a limitless source of sauces, meats, seasonings, eggs, and veggies which do not demand higher corn syrup additives and carbohydrate high sugar making a lot of tasting meals.

Chapter 7
How Are Ketogenic
Diets' Done Right'

Let's fast discuss the way they work.

Overview of Ketosis Simply, organs, our body, brain, and muscles can utilize either ketones or glucose for fuel. It is the performance of the liver and pancreas (primarily) to regulate which fuel source and they also clearly show a strong bias toward rolling with glucose.

Sugar is the' preferred' fuel since it is derived in abundance from the diet plan and easily available easily from liver and muscle mass retailers. Ketones have to get synthesized by the liver; though the liver can readily synthesize glucose through a procedure known as gluconeogenesis which makes use of amino acids (protein) or any other metabolic intermediaries) also.

Bbeta-hydroxybutyrate, or acetoacetate (ketones) do not come from the diet plan. The liver synthesizes it just under duress; as a measure in conditions of serious glucose deprivation such as starvation. For the liver to be confident that ketones would be the order of the morning, many ailments have to be met:

Blood glucose should fall under 50mg/dl

Low blood glucose must lead to Insulin that is low and elevated Glucagon

Liver glycogen should be minimal or' empty'

An ample source of gluconeogenic substrates mustn't be for sale At this time it is essential to point out it is not, in fact, a question of being' in' or' out' of ketosis; we do not also completely operate on ketones, or not.

It is a careful and gradual transition so that the human brain is evenly and constantly fuelled... ideally. Ketones Must be manufactured in amounts that are small from blood sugar levels of approximately 60mg/dl. We think about ourselves in ketosis when there are better levels of ketones than sugar in the blood.

The truth is that the majority of people especially industry trainers have had a normal intake of glucose for a great couple of years, at least. The liver is absolutely effective at creating ketones however the extremely effective gluconeogenic pathways are in a position to keep low normal blood sugar above the ketogenic threshold.

Couple with the reality that a lot of individuals are a minimum partly insulin resistant and elevated fasting insulin (upper end of the standard range, anyway). The little quantity of blood sugar from gluconeogenesis induces adequate insulin discharge to blunt the production and glucagon output of ketones.

Unexpected glucose deprivation is going to have the consequence, hunger, of lethargy, initially, weakness, etc in many individuals - until ketosis is attained.

And Ketosis won't be covered until the liver is made to stop with gluconeogenesis and begin creating ketones. So long as dietary protein is enough then the liver is going to continue producing glucose and never ketones. That is the reason no carb, high protein diet programs aren't ketogenic.

What's Great About Ketosis?

If the body changes to running mainly on ketones a selection of extremely cool things happens:

Lipolysis (bodyfat breakdown) is considerably increased

Muscle catabolism (muscle loss) is considerably reduced

Energy levels are looked after in a stable and high state

Subcutaneous material (aka' water retention') is removed when we are in ketosis the body is by using body fat to fuel everything. As a result, we are not breaking down the muscle to offer glucose.

That is, the muscle has been spared since it is absolutely nothing to offer; extra fat is all of the body requires (well, to a significant extent). For the dieter what this means is considerably less muscle loss than what is achievable on every other diet. Make sense?

As a bonus, ketones yield just seven calories a gram. This is much higher compared to the identical mass of sugar but considerably fewer (twenty-two %, in fact) compared to the nine caloric g of extra fat from whence it came. We love metabolic inefficiencies this way. They mean we can eat more though the body does not get the calories.

Often cooler is the fact that ketones can't be switched back again to oily acids; the entire body excretes excess in urine! There'll be rather a fall in muscle mass glycogen, minimal aldosterone and minimal Insulin all equate to substantial excretion of extra and intra cellular solution. For us that means tough, defined muscularity and fast, results that are visible.

Concerning energy, the brain in fact Really loves ketones and so we often really feel great in ketosis - clear-headed, positive and alert. Plus simply because there is not a lack of extra fat to provide ketones, energy is high at all times. Generally, you will sleep much less and wake to be more rejuvenated when in ketosis.

To do it Right

From whats stated earlier, you will realize that to enter into ketosis: Carbohydrate consumption must be nil; Zero!

Protein intake needs to be low - twenty-five % of calories in a maximum

Fat should account for 75%+ of energy with lower insulin (due to 0 carbs) and calories at, or even below maintenance, the nutritional fat can't be deposited with adipose cells.

The reduction in protein usually means that gluconeogenesis will rapidly confirm inadequate to keep blood glucose and also if the entire body wants it or not, there is always all of the damned extra fat to burn up.

The substantial nutritional fat is oxidized for cellular energy in the standard manner but ends up producing a number of Acetyl CoA which go over the capability of the TCA cycle.

The substantial outcome is ketogenesis - synthesis of ketones from the surplus Acetyl CoA. In more lay terms: the fatty intake' forces' ketosis in the entire body. This is the way it's done right'.

You now simply need to throw out what you believed was true about fat. For starters, weight does not' make you fat'. The majority of the info about the evils of saturated fat, particularly, is very disproportionate or even plain wrong anyway; on a ketogenic diet plan, it is doubly inapplicable.

Saturated oils force ketosis fly. And do not worry; the heart is going to be a lot better than fine and the insulin sensitivity won't be reduced (there isn't insulin around in the very first place)!

When in ketosis it is not essential, technically speaking, to keep complete zero carbs or minimal protein. Though it is still better in case you want to reap the best rewards. Also, presuming you are training hard, you'll still choose to adhere to a cyclic ketogenic diet in which you get to consume all the carbs, fresh fruit and whatever else, every single 1 2 days, regardless.

They are most likely restrictive diets you can use if you do not love animal products.

Get out the nutritional almanac and figure out a 20:0:80 protein:carb: fat diet plan. Yeah, boring.

You will find a selection of supplements which help in making Keto diets potent. Nevertheless, a lot of popular supplements will be wasted. Here's an introduction of the key ones:

Al and chromium enhance insulin sensitivity leading to higher glucagon, lower insulin levels, and a fast descent into much deeper ketosis creatine is somewhat of a misuse - at nearly all, thirty % may be used in place by the muscles which, with no glycogen, can't be meaningfully' volumized'.

HMB (in case it works) would/should be a great product for minimizing the catabolic period before ketosis is achieved

Tribulus is great and also comes really recommended as it magnifies the enhanced testosterone output of a ketogenic diet Carnitine in Acetyl-L or L form is a nearly important supplement for Keto Diets.

Glutamine, free-form crucial and branched-chain amino are worthy for post and pre-training. Simply do not overdo the glutamine while it supports gluconeogenesis. L-Carnitine is needed for the development of ketones in the liver.

ECA stack body fat burners are extremely helpful and crucial though do not care about the addition of HCA Flaxseed oil is an excellent but don't assume you require fifty % of the calories from fatty acids. 1 10 % of calories is more than adequate.

Whey Protein is elective - you do not want excessive protein Remember!

A soluble fiber supplement which is noncarbohydrate based is great. But walnuts are much easier.

Chapter 8
How Do You Know
If You're Burning Fat?

Ketosis is a state of fat-burning autopilot in your body. How's this? The fat stored in your body begins to be used as energy to reduce weight, not water or muscle.

Many diets promoted are diets restricting calories. They help you lose weight, but most weight is water and muscle. Little fat stores breakdown.

Here's the calorie-restrictive eating problem. Your metabolism gets slower because your body starts thinking it's starving and has to slow down the calorie loss process. A slow metabolism represents slower weight loss and faster weight gain.

Cyclic ketogenic diet limits carbohydrates. By limiting carbohydrates, but maintaining caloric consumption, your body will have one fuel consumption option. That's fat; that's ketosis. You're turning your fat-burning machine on.

Ketones are sent out of your body, and deep fat loss. How's this happening? The key player is the body's largest internal organ. It's your liver. The liver transforms fat into ketones. Then these ketones are excreted from the body, weight / fat loss. It's a natural process.

Ketones are created in the liver and an efficient body energy source. As these ketones, fatty acids from body fat are created in the liver. Ketones can only occur when the body lacks sugar and glucose.

Carbohydrates contain both substances. Losing weight on a high-carbohydrate diet will always be hard. On the ketogenic diet, sugar and glucose levels are reduced to the point where they are no longer the primary source of fuel to be burned in the bloodstream.

We should take a moment to talk about a few myths surrounding the ketogenic diet and whether it's long-term health. Our bodies can perform ketosis and be healthy. This ketosis state occurs naturally when the body does not use sugar and glucose. Naturally, the human body has no issue in this state. In other words, burning fat is safe.

A simple walk to the drug store can respond quickly. Check your ketosis level using ketone test strips. Simply catch a sample of urine on strips and test for color change. The magic color is a pink to purple result. Check the color scale to see your ketone level in the fat-burning zone.

Using these strips will be your cause of released ketone level. This is the gage you'll understand if you keep your carbohydrate consumption to the required level to promote ketosis. Don't worry if there's no

Dark violet level. Different people have varying rates. Watch the scale, and if you lose weight, you're fine.

Here's a dehydration alert. If you see dark purple, make sure you drink enough water. Sometimes dark-purple indicates dehydration. Make sure the ketogenic plan correctly hydrated.

A mechanism related to ketosis is essential to cyclical ketogenic diet. Restricting carbohydrates and allowing your body to burn fat reserves will help you achieve your weight loss and body contour goals. Get your ketone strips and watch burning start.

Cyclical ketogenic diet is no longer a fad cyclical ketogenic diet. As more individuals see the importance of the diet, the attention it deserves starts. This diet advantages from treating obesity to epilepsy. The nice news is, if you want to lose weight and still enjoy some of those junk foods, you've come to the correct location.

Low-carb diet is a long-term news media "fad." With so many differences on low-carb diet, this eating scheme seems forever in the news. Whether you're a football coach, administrative assistant or high school teacher, the low-carb cyclical ketogenic diet is for you.

It's not the Atkins diet or some variation of the eating plan. Those who benefit most from Atkins plans are those who are not generally intensive about physical activity and may restrict their activity to aerobic exercise like walking 3 times a week.

For those who want to burn fat but maintain muscle mass, the cyclical ketogenic diet plan. This will assist keep intense reorganization exercise programs and strengthen your body.

Yes, use Atkins ' plan to lose weight. The issue with this scheme, though, is you'll also lose water and muscle mass. If you're athletic and want to maintain your physical form, that's not the direction you're going.

The CKD lets you burn the fat and increase the muscle mass that most people want. Scientifically, the more muscle mass you have, the healthier your body and bones will be in future years. You get all this, and a Saturday night you can eat those fun foods. What a settlement.

Will it take some knowledge? Absolutely. It'll take a few weeks for your body to eat this way and fight off carb cravings. Persevere, exercise discipline. Ultimately, you'll win so long-term thinking and a finisher strategy.

All diets and exercise programs are said to work. It's the individuals who choose not to work. Learning to think long-term with your mental attitude together will be key to your diet success.

We must all learn to work smarter, not harder. That's your cyclical ketogenic diet. Simply put, we must understand the big picture and set goals accordingly. Just giving up carbohydrates, working out and watching the fat melt away is not the game plan here. Follow this chapter's logical plan and accomplishment.

There'll be some math here, but hold on, and we'll get through it. Your lean weight is the first calculation to create. Naturally, this won't be your complete body weight. Let's take an instance weighing 200 pounds.

Assuming, your body fat is 20%, your lean body mass weight will definitely be 160 pounds. Protein calories are 640 magic. That's obtained by multiplying your body mass learning times 4. Remember amount: 640.

Your calorie equilibrium should arrive, you guessed, fat. The irony here is eating fat to begin the fat-burning furnace. You have to get used to that. Many advantages come in eating this way.

You'll feel fuller as fat moves through the digestive system slowly. Facially, fatty food also tastes good. There are also reduced glucose features that reduce insulin and efficiently kick in fat-burning hormones.

Now you may have a response everybody wishes. What's fat consumption?

More math: begin with a 500 calorie shortage from your calories. Here's the number. It's 15 times your weight. This would imply about 3,000 calories to retain and 2500 to begin losing fat from our 200 pound instance above.

So, 2500 less is our 1860 protein calories, which amounts to about 206 grams of fat per day. That's it. That's eating plan for the weekday diet. Something to consider. As time goes on, and your diet well, you may need to limit more calories. Remember to cut fat calories, not protein.

Recently, there has been much debate as to whether the cyclical ketogenic diet can long be maintained. The debate generally focuses on reduced carbohydrate imbalance. The diet plan involves 36-hour carbohydrate loading, typically weekends.

You're free to consume carbohydrates. It's two things. First, a weekend dieter incentive; weekend pizza. Second, it replenishes lost carbohydrates, which helps balance the system and provide energy for the next cycle.

Perhaps another question should be asked. And what's a healthy eating issue?

Depriving yourself of pizza and ice cream, products we know are not great for us, regarded bad.

If cyclical ketogenic diet can assist to balance good blood pressure and stabilize blood sugar through the workout stage, and help burn fat, then its high time you look at it as a good alternative to what is marketed as healthy eating. This eating plan has more long-term benefits than disadvantages.

Chapter 9
The Science Behind Ketosis

When the body is fueled entirely by fat, it enters a state known as "Ketosis," which is a natural state for the body. Once all the sugars and unhealthy fats are taken out of the body through the first 2 or 3 weeks, the body is free to run on healthy ones.

There are many possible benefits of ketosis related to accelerated weight loss, health or performance. In certain situations such as type 1 and type 2 diabetes, excessive ketosis can become extremely dangerous.

Ketosis state is achieved when the level of ketones increases dramatically in blood flow. These ketones are basically chemicals that are formed when the liver begins using fat for energy sources. Why would the liver begins using fat instead of sugar for physiological energy requirements? You might ask.

The solution to this is pretty straightforward. When you start hungry your body then the amount of sugar will decrease dramatically and will ultimately perish within the body.

Now the liver would turn to proteins from the tissues for meeting the energy requirements but finally these stored proteins may also perish and now there is nothing left except for stored fats when it comes to supplying energy to the entire body. Hence, the liver will start burning these fats for fulfilling the minimum energy requirements of the body.

It's at this stage that ketones are formed. Basically they are a by-product of their lipid metabolic pathway following the fat is converted into energy. It is very important to mention that many specialist esteem Ketosis or Ketone bodies as the crisis reaction of the body into some carbohydrate deficient diet.

Therefore it would suffice to state that ketosis diet is not recommended by the vast majority of experts except for under extreme circumstances. But this view is coming into question and many doctors assert that Ketosis diet may indeed work so far as weight loss is concerned.

Hence ketosis diet or ketogenic Diet, to be medically precise, is a very low carbohydrate diet with emphasis on moderate protein and high fat nutrition. Conventionally, it has been used as a treatment for diabetes and several physicians have supported its claim of being helpful in weight loss.

The diet operates in similar facets to starvation with an important twist. In the latter, the body is deprived of all diet for several days while depending upon juices, drinks or water to get getting by but when it comes to Ketosis diet, the body is forced to burn fat instead of carbohydrate for meeting its energy condition.

In the absence of carbohydrate, the liver can burn fat and turn it into fatty acids and ketones or ketone bodies. Obviously, to accomplish the ends of ketosis diet, all carbohydrate rich foods such as cereal grains, sugar, specific vegetables etc. need to be eliminated from diet.

In addition to it, naturally occurring foods like eggs, meat, fish, which contain nominal or nearly no carbohydrate, ought to be consumed in abundance during meals.

Most times, when we hear of a diet that puts the body in a state of ketosis, we are scared to know that ketosis is a possibly hazardous blood sugar imbalance arising from low carbohydrate high protein diet. Ketosis results from burning glucose to burning ketones.

Glucose arises from carbohydrates, the body's first energy metabolization option. Ketones are used for energy when there is inadequate glucose (carbohydrate) in the bloodstream.

Clinically mentioned, "Ketosis is a disease in which blood concentrations of ketones (ketone bodies) are elevated. Ketones are formed when glycogen stored in the liver are out of supply. Ketones are used for energy purposes.

Ketones are tiny carbon fragments produced by fat storage breakdowns. Ketosis can be a severe disease if ketone concentrations go too high." The body can also get all its fat and protein energy.

An early 1900s ketogenic diet is a high-fat, low-carbohydrate diet. The body, after a ketogenic diet, moves from a carb-burning machine to a fat-burning machine.

Weight loss results.

The Atkins plan may be the best-known ketonic diet, where ketosis is intentionally accomplished through high-fat protein and low-carbohydrate diet. According to the Atkins program, adequate urine surveillance will keep ketosis within secure boundaries and the dieter can attain an ideal body weight without experiencing unbearable hunger.

The high fat content discourages most patients from following an Atkins-type diet. Surgery decreases digestive gastric juice, and many patients do not tolerate high-fat foods.

Experts are split on health danger vs. ketogenic diet in general population (. Some specialists say it's hazardous because if ketone concentrations are not controlled correctly, kidney strain may happen, and a substantial loss of urine-excreted calcium may trigger osteoporosis or kidney stones.

The proponents of a ketogenic diet quote human evolution in their reasoning that we have long been a hunter-gatherer species in a ketogenic state. Documented studies suggest that after 2-4 weeks of adaptation, ketosis doesn't influence human physical endurance.

Some studies go so far that people don't necessarily need elevated carbohydrate intakes to substitute depleted glycogen shops for energy.

Patients should work intimately with their bariatric center to create a particular lifestyle and diet program for recovery and obesity. While many see the main weight loss surgery objective as weight loss to enhance physical appearance, the greater objective is health, energy, and longevity.

Chapter 10
The Science Behind 7 Keto DHEA

7 Keto DHEA littered in weight loss headlines. Although it explains the health advantages of 7 Keto DHEA, there was little explanation as to what it does.

7 Keto DHEA is a DHEA metabolite, known for improving the impacts of aging on many body functions. Since 7 Keto DHEA does not alter into estrogens or testosterone, its parent is 100% secure.

There are signs that 7 Keto DHEA helps the body decrease weight by imitating thyroid hormones, causing the body to generate more heat, burning more calories without doing anything. This implies, to some extent, thyroid enzymes can be deemed thermogenic.

Increasing IL-2 manufacturing in human lymphocytes enables the immune system better. IL-2 is the primary T-helper cytokine controller that helps activate the immune system for invading pathogens. It reduces cortisol. Cortisol is a stress-related hormone, besides serious mental disorders and aging.

Using 7 Keto DHEA increases the body's resting metabolic rate. RMR (resting metabolism rate) is the little calories the body needs to maintain its normal functions, including breathing, digesting food, circulating blood, etc.

By increasing the RMR, your body will naturally burn additional calories per day, exceeding your calorie intake. Your body will start consuming your back, stomach, thighs, and other body components.

A constant natural weight loss results.

7 Keto DHEA supplement is regarded unlike some other metabolism amplifier as it is natural in the body.

Benefits of 7 Keto Supplement

There are many nutritional products on the market, and only few can articulate. In recent years, 7-keto's natural weight loss characteristics have endorsed recognition. However, weight loss isn't the sole benefit of this supplement.

Some of the advantages include: Enhance metabolism Its primary role is to boost your metabolism so you can burn more fat while you rest. Your RMR should be enhanced to dissolve your thighs and stomach away from fat and clean.

One latest research evaluated 7 Keto supplement's capacity to obtain better immune objective in older respondents. Accordingly, the study disclosed that after only four weeks, respondents obtained elevated white blood cell concentrations, were able to brawl disease quicker, and acquired cells to boost the body's immune system.

Slows aging

Similar to human growth hormones and IGF-1, natural amounts of 7 Keto decrease after reaching a point. The research revealed that 7 Keto supplement could help slow the aging process and even invert the aging process if taken early.

Improves Cholesterol

Studies showed that 25 mg7-keto daily was adequate to significantly improve HDL cholesterol levels and lower LDL levels. Some participants also witness that 7 Keto DHEA reduced their cholesterol level by thirty points in six weeks, which is sufficient to significantly reduce the risk of heart related health problems.

Weight loss and 7-Keto-DHEA

7-Keto-DHEA has been acclaimed as a stronger and safer alternative to DHEA for anti-aging and weight loss.

As the hormone DHEA's active metabolite, 7-Keto-DHEA is multiples times potent than DHEA to improve thermogenesis by stimulating production of enzyme in the liver in the absence of androgenic side effects like hair loss, benign prostatic hyperplasia, and virilization. Many modern users prize the supplement for its accelerating effect on diet and exercise weight loss.

Young people usually have more muscle, fewer wrinkles, and an easier time losing fat as compared to older people. As hormone levels decline and age sets in, aging symptoms appear as fat accumulation and lean muscle loss.

Hormone supplementation can reduce or eliminate these problems, but substances like DHEA testosterone also cause numerous androgenic effects that contribute to high blood pressure and cancer.

Using 7-Keto-DHEA allows users to fight aging effects while avoiding the side effects associated with other hormonal supplements.

How it relates to metabolism Weight loss is normally difficult to maintain because, in response to reduced food intake, metabolism slows rapidly. This process, known as the metabolic set-point, can prevent many individuals from ever seeing much result from their diet and exercise efforts.

7-Keto-DHEA keeps the set point down, allowing individuals to keep losing weight throughout their diet and exercise programs. Rather than directly causing weight loss, it dramatically improves body response to consistent efforts over time.

Effects on Thermogenesis

Many weight loss supplements, including caffeine, work by increasing basal body temperature and effectively burning away fat. 7-Keto also accomplishes this; enhancing the activity of enzymes in the liver increases thermogenesis, but without increasing blood pressure or androgen levels.

This means 7-Keto-DHEA is much safer for long-term weight loss regimens, which are more likely to last.

Other Weight Loss Benefits 7 Keto DHEA also speeds weight loss by raising T3 levels, a metabolism-involved thyroid hormone. Professional athletes often supplement pure, exogenous T3, but 7-Keto-

DHEA rises T3 safely and naturally. Studies have demonstrated that the parent hormone, DHEA, eats more without increasing its weight.

One research has shown that animal feed consumption in command should be halved to produce the same body weight changes encountered by DHEA cattle with a standard diet. 7-Keto-DHEA also has an impressive safety profile; it is usually suggested for tiny doses of 100-200 mg per day but big amounts have been tested without causing health issues.

Researchers say that a huge dose of 140,000 mg 7-Keto-DHEA can leave a person with liver values and ordinary blood chemistries.

Instead of being an independent component in quick and simple weight loss, 7-Keto-DHEA is a reliable way of speeding up weight loss in combination with exercise and low-calory diet.

Persons of all ages can profit from even small weight loss, and without adverse adverse effects 7-Keto-DHEA will make it simpler to accomplish. The person may obtain all these health advantages in one package instead of using individual thermogenesis supplements, thyroid stimulation and lean muscle gain.

7-Keto-DHEA plays a key role in many body procedures as the natural active metabolite of the hormone DHEA. 7-Keto-DHEA concentrations decrease throughout life, but supplementation can restore levels. Users obtain classic 7-keto advantages, with reduced cortisol, better immune function, weight loss and retention.

How 7-Keto-DHEA works with 7-Keto-DHEA improves the rate of weight loss, mainly by raising thermogenesis body temperature. Thermogenesis also increases with additional supplements like DHEA, caffeine and éphedrine, but these drugs often have unwanted side impacts, such as elevated blood pressure.

Improving thermogenesis without side effects is one of the main advantages of 7-Keto. For its benefits 7-Keto can be used without causing toxicity even in very big dosages. One research discovered that animals with the equivalent of 40,000 mg per day, about 200-400 times the recommended daily normal dose of 100 or 200 mg, had no ill impacts.

The enhanced 7-keto-DHEA metabolic rate enables nutritioners to continue to benefit long after their diets are started. In place of a slow metabolism induced by a low-calorie diet, consumers experience constant metabolic increase and prevent weight loss on a plateau.

Therefore,7-keto improves T3 thyroid hormone. Some supplements for weight loss, such as l-tyrosine, boost fat burning by raising T3 but ultimately collapse with use. In comparison, 7-Keto maintains a elevated T3 level in customers, enabling them to continually pour pounds.

Scientists have observed that this increase in T3 stays within a secure and normal range, enabling consumers to harvest the benefits of increased T3 while avoiding too much falling.

7-Keto-DHEA is not a miracle weight loss supplement, but is a miracle that causes consumers to lose fat effortlessly. However, the main advantages of decreased cortisol, improved T3 and enhanced thermogenesis coupled with diet and workout are significantly simplified.

7 The advantages of Keto include reducing cortisol, which allows people to train harder and more often during regimen. This is just another way 7-Keto-DHEA makes weight loss easier.

7-Keto-DHEA also increases body insulin use along with its other benefits, preventing increase in fat. 7-Keto includes more elements of dietary fitness than other contemporary weight loss supplements.

Wherefore DHEA may be important in 7 keto dhea or dehydroepiandrosterone form, a steroid that is often naturally made complemented by athletes, enables fat loss, muscle gain, power increase and libido to enhance testosterone concentrations.

The average person who wanted to be more athletic, lose weight or gain muscle discovered that they were able to do the same thing gained huge public attraction.

Many fitness supplements used DHEA as part of their point of sale during the 1990s and early 2000s. Many studies have detailed the impacts of DHEA on all the athletic activities listed above and also several surprising beneficial advantages.

Increased production of insulin, better sex driving, enhanced mood, enhanced memory, greater concentrations of "healthy" HDL cholesterol, and multiple immune advantages. In fact, in latest years, a number of DHEA supplements have emerged on the racks in your local vitamin store, demonstrating potential damage to DHEA.

DHEA has shown that certain gender hormones— multiple strong androgenic and estrogens — are higher. These sex hormones control a number of significant body procedures and cause all kinds of unwanted side effects, such as surplus face hair (male and female), mood swings, hyperglycemia, and even carcinoma.

Why 7 Keto DHEA better?

Fortunately, researchers created a nearly identical molecule of DHEA without its propensity to discard the natural equilibrium of the body's hormones. It is a natural metabolite of DHEA known as 7 Keto DHEA. This implies that ingesting DHEA does not cause DHEA to cause many of the desirable advantages you want.

The body metabolizes DHEA into 7 Keto DHEA and a number of hormone enhancers. By pre-metabolizing DHEA in 7 Keto DHEA and throwing out unnecessary compounds, scientists can generate precise same impacts as DHEA without any side impacts.

What are some of 7 Keto DHEA's proven benefits?

Fat reduction* Increased energy production* Immune benefits— increase in anti-viral antibodies* Effective muscle and weight loss treatment for HIV or waste disease patients* Improves HDL cholesterol, reduces risk of heart disease, heart attack, and stroke A few important details on these benefits.

First of all, weight loss results require at least 200 mg of fat per day. That's just the minimum-some people take up to 1400 mg daily depending on their weight loss goals.

Many supplement companies sell 7 Keto DHEA capsules containing only 50 to 100 mg each, requiring a daily minimum of two or four pills. Companies don't tell you this, because taking 7 Keto DHEA at the daily dosage required is quite expensive. 7 Keto DHEA actually costs more than pure DHEA as a supplement.

Increased energy production can also come at a cost. The reason why energy production is increased is linked to 7 Keto DHEA use as a weight loss product. DHEA does two things related to energy production: facilitates the body's metabolization of fats into energy, making the body less efficient in burning fat.

This makes the body produce more energy by burning exponentially more fat. This is great if you have a lot of fat, but if you don't have any fat on your body, 7 Keto DHEA can be a dangerous product. By reducing the body's efficiency, you can actually experience energy reduction.

Regardless of these details, studies showing 7 Keto DHEA's efficacy in these areas are unassailable.

Some other DHEA benefits This list includes a number of proven DHEA benefits for which 7 Keto DHEA studies have not yet been conducted:* Decreases lupus symptoms such as rashes, anemia, arthritis, and heart, lung, or kidney problems* Better mood* Increases libido, better sex drive* Normalizes blood sugar, prevents diabetes*

Anti-aging-reverses tissue deterioration While it only makes sense to have similar benefits, one should be wary of advertising websites or products that make claims of these benefits. Especially the heightened libido/sex drive claim is somewhat dubious, as it is not supposed to increase levels of sex hormones.

Dangers of 7-keto DHEA

If you don't have any fat to burn, DHEA can actually decrease your energy levels.

Studies have shown that it can actually decrease blood levels of sex hormone. This result is credible because it doesn't increase them like pure DHEA.

Chapter 11
Fat And Protein Ratio In
A Ketogenic Diet

The ketogenic diet, colloquially known as the keto diet, is a favorite diet that contains excessive quantities of fat, low carbohydrate, and adequate protein. It is likewise called a Low Carb High Fat (LCHF) diet and a reduced carb diet plan. It was mainly formulated for the therapy of epilepsy which didn't respond to pills for the disease.

The traditional ketogenic diet plan has a "fat" to some "combination of protein and carbohydrates" ratio of 4:1.

The overall day calorie malfunction of the ketogenic diet plan can be as follows:

60-80 % of calories at fat

20-25 % from proteins

5-10 % coming from carbohydrates

The ratio of the meals in a ketogenic diet plan is developed to assist the body induce and keep a state of ketosis.

Nevertheless, the ketogenic landscape has enhanced significantly each in its implementation and application. Even though the classical ketogenic diet plan is still extensively used these days, it has today formed the grounds for the improvement of numerous alternative ketogenic protocols.

Ketogenic diets generally encourage the intake of approximately twenty to fifty grams of carbohydrates each day. Protein use is reasonable and usually depends on things like the gender, level and activity levels of the person. Basically, the general calorie of the diet is healthy largely depending on the quantity of ingested fat.

The Protein and Fat Ratios in a Ketogenic Diet Increased good fat usage will be the primary target of the ketogenic diet plan. Furthermore, the objective is maintaining the state of ketosis all the time, therefore, allowing the body to take a lot of body fat for fuel.

The human body digests body fat and protein differently. Extra fat could well be the body 's very best supply of energy and also in a state of ketosis, the body can use dietary fat and body fat every bit as properly.

Generally, fats have quite limited impact on blood sugar and insulin production in the body. Nevertheless, protein affects both these levels if consumed in a lot beyond what the body requires.

Approximately fifty-six % of the surplus ingested protein is changed to sugar. This has got the outcome of upsetting the ketosis state of much burning as an outcome of the entire body responding to the sugar produced out of the protein breakdown.

Based on the sort and supply of ingested fats, a higher fat diet can be far healthier. Decreasing carb consumption and also increasing the consumption of more saturated fat from mainly medium-chain fatty acids will significantly enhance your body 's fat profile.

The ketogenic diet improves HDL (good) cholesterol levels while simultaneously decreases triglyceride levels. These 2 factors are the primary markers for cardiovascular disease.

A ratio of under 2.0 in the Triglyceride-to-HDL ratio means you are doing well. Nevertheless, the better this ratio is usually to 1.0 or even lower, the healthier the heart.

This particular sort of fat profile is related to improved protection against heart attacks and other cardiovascular issues.

Intake of improved lean protein in the lack of sufficient quantities of fat in the eating plan can trigger "rabbit starvation." Rabbit starvation is a problem where there is an inadequate quantity of fat. This particular problem is observed in diets which mainly include lean proteins.

Among the main symptoms of rabbit starvation is diarrhea. Diarrhea could become really serious and may result in death.

This usually occurs within the very first three days to seven days of pure lean protein diet programs. If sufficient quantities of oils aren't used in the succeeding days, diarrhea can worsen and could result in possible death and dehydration.

Chapter 12
Is The Keto Diet Plan Safe For You?

You should be mindful the entire body uses sugars in the type of glycogen to run. The keto diet which is very restricted in sugar forces the body to use body fat as fuel rather than sugar, since it doesn't get adequate sugar.

When the entire body doesn't get adequate sugar for fuel, the liver is made to change the accessible extra fat in ketones which are worn by the body as fuel - thus the word ketogenic.

This particular diet plan is a high-fat diet with reasonable quantities of protein. Based on your carbohydrate consumption the body gets to a state of ketosis in under a week and stays there. As extra fat is needed rather than sugar for fuel in the entire body, the losing weight is remarkable with no supposed restriction of calories.

The keto diet is so that you must try to get 60 75 % of the daily calories from fat, 15 30 % coming from protein and just 5-10 % from carbs. This typically means that you can consume just 20 50 grams of carbs in one day.

The diet plan is a high-fat diet which is fairly much like Atkins. Nevertheless, there is an increased focus on fat, usually' good' fats.

You can additionally get an entire selection of snacks that are intended for keto followers. As you can see because of this list, fruits are restricted. You can have sugar fruits that are low in a small amount (mostly berries) but must forego the favorite fruits as these are almost all sweet-tasting or starchy.

This particular eating habit has no grains of any type, starchy veggies as potatoes (and most tubers), without high sugar or sweets, no bread & cakes, absolutely no beans & lentils, absolutely no pasta, without burgers and pizza & hardly any alcohol. And also this means no espresso with tea or milk with milk - in fact, milk-based desserts and ice-creams and no milk.

A number of these have workarounds as you can get carbohydrate-free pizza and pasta, you can have cauliflower rice and today there are also restaurants that focus on keto aficionados.

If you are thinking if this diet is secure, the proponents and those individuals who have achieved the weight loss goals will definitely agree it is healthy.

Type two diabetes patients on the keto diet eating plan might be in a position to decrease the medications

Several good things about people suffering from cancer Aside from the very first 4, there is not adequate evidence to allow for the effectiveness or usually for other illnesses as a great deal more research is needed within the long term.

Will be there any side-effects from this diet?

Once you primarily launch the keto diet, you can experience what is referred to as keto flu. These signs might not happen in most individuals and in most cases begin a couple of days after getting on the diet plan, when the body is in a state of ketosis.

Carbohydrate and sugar cravings

These could get as much as a week to diminish as the body get used to the new diet program. You can additionally suffer from other issues if you begin the keto diet plan - you might find you have increased urination, therefore it is essential to keep yourself very well hydrated.

You might, in addition, suffer from keto breath when the body reaches ideal ketosis and also you can utilize a mouthwash or even clean the teeth a bit more regularly. Often the unwanted side effects are brief and once the body acclimatizes on the latest diet, these can disappear.

The same as every other diet plan which restricts foods in particular types, the keto diet isn't with no risks. As you are not meant to eat numerous vegetables and fruits, beans and other foods and lentils, you can suffer from lack of several important nutrients.

Since the diet is loaded with fats that are saturated and also, in case you indulge in the' bad' fat, you can have higher cholesterol amounts upping the risk of heart problems.

In the long-range, the keto diet program could additionally result in a lot of food deficiencies since you can't consume grains, many vegetables, and fruits and overlook fiber as likewise vital vitamins, minerals, antioxidants, and phytonutrients and other items.

You can be afflicted by intestinal distress, lowered bone density (other sources and no dairy of calcium) and liver and kidney problems (the diet puts extra pressure on both organs).

In case you are inclined to forego the usual dietary staples and are really sharp to reduce weight, you might be enticed to check out the keto diet plan.

The 1 problem with the keto diet is poor patient compliance due to the carbohydrate restriction, so you need to make sure that you can abide with the food choices. In case you just think it is too tough to follow, you can go on an edition of the revised keto diet which provides more carbs.

Nevertheless, the keto diet is certainly good at assisting you to shed weight. Based on a recently available study, a lot of the obese patients followed had been effective in slimming down. Any problems they faced were transient.

When you don't have any substantial health issues except for obesity and also have been unsuccessful in slimming down following any standard diet, the keto eating plan could a practical choice.

You should be absolutely motivated to shed the excess weight and also be ready to begin a restricted diet plan as specified. Even in case, you have any health issues, you can get your doctor 's advice and a nutritionist 's assistance and go on this particular diet plan.

Yet another study which was performed for an extended time demonstrated that happening the keto diet is advantageous in dieting and results in decreased cholesterol levels with a reduction in the bad cholesterol and a rise in the very good cholesterol.

Many physicians and nutritionists are agreed the keto diet is great for weight reduction with the short term. As for the long term, more experiments are needed. Do keep in your mind that obesity isn't an apt option as it has your own risk of health issues.

For a lot of people, a keto diet is incredibly secure. Nevertheless, you will find specific people who have to have special care and consult with the doctors before taking such a diet plan. All those taking medicines for diabetes. Dosage may have to be adjusted as blood glucose goes down with a low carb diet.

All those taking medicines for high blood pressure. The dosage might have been modified as blood pressure level goes down with a low carb diet plan.

Those people who are breastfeeding shouldn't go on a really strict low carb diet as the body can lose approximately 30 g of carbs each day via the milk. Thus, have no less than 50 g of carbs each day while breastfeeding.

Those with kidney disease must talk to the doctors before creating a keto diet.

Typical Concerns With a Keto Diet

Not being ready to achieve ketosis. Be sure you are refusing to eat far too much protein and there are no hidden carbs in the packaged foods which you eat.

Eating the wrong fat types like the extremely refined polyunsaturated corn and soybean oils.

Symptoms of a "keto flu", like feeling light-headed, brain fog, fatigue, headaches, dizziness, and constipation. When in ketosis, the entire body is likely to excrete more sodium. In case one isn't getting plenty of sodium from the diet plan, symptoms of a keto flu may seem.

This is fast dealt with by consuming two cups of broth (with additional salt) each day. When you work out vigorously or the sweat rate is excessive, you might have to include back again a lot of sodium.

Dawn impact. Normal fasting blood sugars are a bit less compared to hundred mg/dl and nearly all individuals in ketosis will do this level in case they are not diabetic. Nevertheless, in some individuals fasting blood sugars often rise, particularly in the early morning, while holding a keto diet plan.

This is known as the "dawn effect" and it is because of the standard circadian increase in early morning cortisol (stress hormone) which induces the liver making glucose.

When this occurs, see to it that you are not ingesting extreme protein at dinner and never too near bedtime. Poor sleep and stress could additionally result in higher cortisol levels. In case you are insulin resistant, you may even need more hours to achieve ketosis.

Minimal sports performance. Keto-adaptation generally takes approximately 4 weeks. During which, rather than doing intense training or workouts, switch to something that is less vigorous. Following the

adaptation time period, athletic performance generally comes back to normal or more effective, particularly for endurance sports.

Keto-rash isn't a typical complication of the diet plan. Likely causes include generation of acetone (a kind of ketone) in the sweat which irritates the skin or nutrient deficiencies like minerals or protein. Shower right after exercise and ensure you consume nutrient-dense whole food items.

Ketoacidosis. This is a really uncommon condition that happens when blood ketone amounts exceed fifteen mM. A formulated keto diet doesn't cause ketoacidosis. Specific circumstances for example type one diabetes, being on medicines with SGLT 2 inhibitors for type two diabetes, or breastfeeding needs additional caution.

Symptoms include lethargy, vomiting, nausea, and fast shallow breathing. cases that are mild can be resolved using baking soda mixed with diluted apple or orange juice. Serious symptoms require prompt medical attention.

This is something of some controversy. Although there haven't been some experiments indicating any undesirable long-range negative effects of getting on a keto diet, most experts today think the body might create a "resistance" on the profits of ketosis unless 1 frequently cycles in & from it. Additionally, eating an extremely high-fat diet in the long-term might not be appropriate for those body types.

When you are competent to produce more than 0.5 mM of ketones in the blood on a regular basis, it is time to begin reintroducing carbs back into the diet plan.

Rather than consuming just 20 50 g of carbs/day, you might wish to boost it to 100 150 g on those carb feeding days. Usually, 2 3 times a week is going to be enough. Ideally, this is additionally accomplished on strength training days where you really boost the protein intake.

Chapter 13
Keto Diet And Plant Based Eating

Keto diet, a common high-fat, low-carb diet pattern, is intended to ketose your body to burn fat rather than sugar. Advocates claim more energy, weight loss, and other health advantages.

Meanwhile, plant-based eating can improve your heart and atmosphere. The ketotarian diet combines both, meaning adherents reduce carbs and eliminate meat.

Examples of foods on the highly restrictive scheme, including lots of eggs, avocados, and coconut oil.

Keto is based on a low-carb diet that limits foods such as bread, grains, cereals, pasta, beans, starchy veggies, sugar, most fruits, and other sweeteners. Usually eating more butter, red meat, and cheese. But reducing animal products is also common, as a plant-based diet has well-known advantages to heart health and planet protection.

So what's your choice?

The ketogenic diet offers the advantages of ketosis— transition to burning fat instead of sugar— but without the health and environmental hazards of any animal goods.

What you can eat?

Avocados, vegetables, wild fish, olives, coconuts, nuts, seeds, fresh seafood, eggs and ghee (clear butter).

"You can really get all your nutrients into a ketotarian diet," your body's fundamental rules are listening eating when you're hungry until you are satisfied) and mixing non-starchy veggies and healthy fats.

But other health specialists said diet is unnecessarily restrictive and unsustainable. "I worry that the rules are not clear enough and could trigger unwanted anxiety about otherwise healthy foods such as fruits and vegetables other than greens

Here's what some typical ketotary meals look like and how healthy they really are. Egg-o-cado, avocados and their mixture are all popular keto products, particularly for vegetarians.

It's nutrient-dense, about 17 grams of protein, 34 grams of fat, and 13 grams of carbs. Eggs are a great source of potassium and folate, particularly from free-range chickens, packaging B vitamins and lutein that are great for your eyes.

Both eggs and avocados also have plenty of vitamin E for your immune system.

Creamed kale

Creamed kale greens are a nice ketotarian replacement in coconut milk instead of dairy. Kale is well-known as a powerhouse with vitamin K, vitamin A, and vitamin C. It's also high in fiber that's great for digestion and can assist you feel fuller.

Coconut milk is high in potassium, vital to muscle health. It's also high in iron, needed for your red blood cells and associated with good energy levels. This dish is about 1,000 calories, primarily from avocado oil and coconut milk.

(Kale is about 33 calories for one cup.) It has 23 grams of protein and 40 grams of carbs. The dish also includes about 100 grams of fat, 75% of which is saturated fat. This can assist adherents get or remain in ketosis, and latest study suggests that saturated fat may be better for health than earlier assumed.

Too much saturated fat has long been correlated with increasing cholesterol concentrations. It can also trigger cholesterol buildup in your arteries, increasing danger of heart disease.

Pesto zoodle bowls

A "zoodle" is a low-carb pasta substitute produced with zucchini. Low-carb zucchini "noodles" provide plenty of vitamin C, which is essential for healthy immune systems. They can also safeguard against heart disease and hypertension. Pesto, spinach with basil, walnuts and olive oil is nutrient-filled: magnesium, calcium, potassium, vitamins A, C, and K.

This dish has little protein, about 8 grams in total, though components vary. It's also low-carbon with about 15 grams of carbohydrates. Again, here's a lot of saturated fat from olive oil and nuts, which is something to remember if you're at danger for heart problems.

Roasted cauliflower with olives, hot sauce,and lemons

Roasted cauliflower with olives, hot sauce, and lemons Cauliflower steaks are keto-friendly, but low in calories, making it hard to make sure you're eating enough. Cauliflower is a cruciferous vegetable containing fiber, vitamin C and B vitamins.

It also includes choline, and significant brain nutrient. Olives (and olive oil) are high in unsaturated fat, which can be useful for your core as

LDL or "poor" cholesterol reduces. Olives are also calorie-dense, about 59 per 10 olives.

They also have calcium and sodium, significant electrolytes for bone, muscle, and nervous function. Overall, though, the recipe is still low in calories, with about 150 to 200 calories ahead, so it probably won't be enough in itself.

Veggie frittata or scramble Different egg and veggie variants can create reliable, good ketotary meals. Eggs are prevalent to many keto diets, and ketotarian is no exception as they're a good, flexible way to mix distinct veggie combinations into a meal.

But also cholesterol-high eggs. Nutritional studies have shown that eggs can increase bad cholesterol concentrations if you consume too many, recommending no more than three eggs a day. For veggies, for instance, almost any keto-friendly options— olives, zucchini, greens, broccoli, peppers— will go well with eggs. I suggest bell peppers, asparagus, spinach and olives.

Vitamin-packed radishes add a low-carb kick to the keto salads. Radishes are low-carb root vegetable a spicy, with lots of fiber, vitamin C and nutrients. Mixed with snow peas, cucumbers, avocado, oil, and vinegar, they create a high fiber lunch salad.

Cucumber, while mostly water, has potassium and vitamin C. Vitamin B2, K, B1, and B3 are carried to the meal along with folate, which is nice for your blood. Although mostly low-calorie veggies, avocado and oil assist fill the salad, so you get enough to eat.

I also suggest adding coconut aminos — an alternative to sweet and salty soy sauce produced from aged coconut sap mixed with salt. It includes amino acids, protein construction blocks.

Fasting

Fasting may have some promising advantages, but study is preliminary and no substitute for healthy eating. Fasting is the reverse of eating a meal. There is some proof that intermittent fasting — restricting meals to a particular period of time during the day — can have health advantages. It can assist decrease long-term health hazards such as diabetes, cholesterol and obesity.

But going keto can already dip people's energy from relying on sugars to fats. Fasting, also affecting energy and metabolism, can be particularly dangerous on diet.

Plus, despite the potential advantages of fasting, a doctor's monitoring should be introduced as part of a carefully planned system, not saving on groceries.

Chapter 14
Analysing Your Weight Loss Objectives

It's not the simplest diet to follow, though, and these early errors can sabotage your weight-loss objectives.

1 The objective of a ketogenic diet is to force your body to stop burning its favourite fuel — glucose from the carbs you eat — and begin burning fat shops for energy.

The body does this by turning fats into ketones— a condition called ketosis. Keto dieters achieve this digestive feat by reducing carbohydrate consumption back. Indeed, keto's average daily objective is 20 grams of net carbs.

But to do it right, you don't just imagine your carb consumption. "If you're a ketogenic diet beginner, counting carbs is a must to prevent future frustration. Track your diet with a wellness app or just use old-fashioned paper and pen.

What you're learning may surprise you. "You may wear' carb-blinders,' meaning you don't know how many carbohydrates you consume in a day,"

2 Keto counter many low-fat diet fads of the 80s and 90s: it actually emphasizes cost.

It's hard to understand because we don't cnsume anything that is pure fat, s" we don't eat a butter stick, a good cup of lard or a spoon of olive oil.

That would be uncomfortable, so we really have a hard time wrapping heads around this notion of ketogenic diet. "To succeed in a keto diet, 60-80% of your diet will be good fats. Nuts, seeds, salmon, butter, bacon and olive oil, are some of the keto-approved choices.

3 You eat too much protein By balancing your macronutrients— fat, protein, carbohydrates— your body has the highest power sources. "The ketogenic diet for' dietary ketosis' is protein – 20%, carbs – 5% and fat – 75%" if you go too high in protein, you're on the Atkins diet and low-carbon.

You'll attain weight loss, but not the health advantages of being in ketosis. "A daily 2,000-calorie keto diet may look like this, according to Harvard Medical School: 165 grams of fat, 40 grams of carbs, and 75 grams of protein. The ratio relies on your particular demands.

4 You don't eat high-quality foods

Many unhealthy foods readily fulfill high-fat low-carbon requirements. That doesn't imply you can eat them freely. "An enormous advantage of pursuing a keto diet is that with grain removal, the vast bulk of processed food is removed.'

Unfortunately, poor-quality milk, veggies and meat can fill the gap.' Look for healthier, better-quality fat and protein including grass-fed meats and maximum restriction of processed dairy.

5. Your electrolytes don't balance your nutritional requirements. Sodium becomes as critical as magnesium

"One of the main electrolytes lost by urination is Mg - magnesium,", "it's mineral energy that helps you burn fat and lose weight. I suggest avoiding magnesium shortage by remaining well-hydrated. I also recommend adding salt and high-magnesium foods to your day.

Magnesium-high foods include almonds, spinach, avocado, chard. Your daily net carbs can blow the cumulative total. "Add carbs in vegetables,". "You can really miss the ketosis mark here and there with cheese, nuts and seeds."

8 Fiber consumption is too low While focusing on fat, protein and carbs, you should also guarantee adequate fiber. "Often people believe they should eat only ketogenic products like meat and butter," you should make sure you eat enough vegetables as you need fiber.

9 When you eat keto, stack white sugar, honey and traditional sugars.

While many artificial sweeteners provide sweetness without one carb, that doesn't mean you should eat them. "We've demonized sugar—just so— for causing unneeded spikes of insulin," but "many artificial sweeteners do exactly the same thing."

Many keto-eaters quickly lose water after starting this diet. Without glycogen (energy) storage carbs, your body burns through them, dumping all the water they hold. That's early keto diet's "water weight

 12 You skip the survey" The biggest mistake people make is that they neglect to do any meaningful keto diet studies, "they hear about a new fad diet or know someone who has a diet. Otherwise, a total diet may fail.' Based your behaviors on what I heard,' or randomly reading a few sentences, isn't smart about any health-related issue.

Chapter 15
Ketogenic Diet For Treating
Type 1 & 2 Diabetes

For those who have Type 2 diabetes, but the problem is a little different. In Type 1 diabetes the insulin-producing cells from the pancreas - known as beta cells have been destroyed or are unable to make insulin. This is usually the result of autoimmune destruction of the pancreas.

People with insulin resistance (prediabetes) usually go on to develop Type 2 diabetes, that's the most common form of the disease. In some Type 2 diabetes, the problem really is that the body doesn't make insulin at the right time or in the ideal amount.

If you eat just a small carbohydrate, or if you eat foods that slow down the passing of high-carbohydrate foods through your digestive tract, then maybe your pancreas can keep up. Or perhaps it can't and your blood glucose remains high with fasting blood sugars at 126 mg/dL (7 mmol/L) or even higher.

Type 2's demand to check your blood sugar level to know whether low-fat diets may work for them. Occasionally a mainly meat diet causes allergic reactions which increase blood sugar levels even more than eating a lot of carbohydrate, and sometimes a mostly meat diet works just fine.

Nearly no-carb, however, is nearly exclusively suitable for people that have MODY or Form 2, and even they need to have some carbohydrate in their eating strategy.

Type 2 diabetes and everyone else, want at least a little bit of carbohydrate in their diet each and every day to generate sugar for "brain fuel"

Usually the absolute lowest amount of carbohydrate from carbohydrate foods daily for any adult is about 40 grams, or 160 to 180 calories (669 to 753 kilojoules). At least this level of carbohydrate must come in the starch stored in plant foods.

The body can turn excess protein into sugar by a procedure which acidifies the urine, but at least a little sugar from food is necessary to assist your brain absorb amino acids from the bloodstream. Even if you are on a ketogenic diet, which is something that you should only try under professional supervision, you need some carbohydrate daily.

As someone who is working hard to ontrol or protect against Type 2 diabetes, one diet you may have learned about is the ketogenic or keto diet program. This diet is a really low carbohydrate diet program composed of approximately.

30% protein, 5% carbohydrates, and 65% dietary fat.

If there is one thing keto diet can do, it's to help control your glucose levels. That being said, there's more to eating nicely than simply controlling your blood sugar.

Let's discuss a few of the main reasons this diet does not always pile up to be as great as it sounds...

1. You are going to be lacking dietary fiber. The first major problem with the ketogenic diet is that'll be lacking in fiber. Almost all veggies are cut from this strategy, fruits and high fibre grains are not permitted which leaves you with primarily fats and protein - two meals containing no fiber at all.

2. You'll be low in energy. Another big issue with the ketogenic diet is you'll be low in energy to carry out your workout program. Your body can only utilize glucose as a fuel supply for very intense exercise and if you aren't taking in carbs, you will not have any glucose available. Therefore, the ketogenic diet is not for everyone who wants to lead an energetic lifestyle with regular workout sessions.

3. You may suffer brain fog. People who are using the ketogenic diet may also find they suffer from brain fog. Again, this is thanks to the fact your brain primarily runs glucose off.

Some people may find following a week or two of using the diet they begin to feel like their mind can switch over to using ketone bodies as a fuel source, but others might never find they begin to feel better.

4. Your antioxidant status will decline. Finally, the previous issue using the ketogenic diet is a result of the shortage of vegetable and fruit content - the antioxidant status is going to sharply decline.

The most dangerous carbohydrate group we don't usually discuss about reducing is sugar. Sugar comprises of simple carbohydrates such as sucrose, fructose, Galactose and simple sugar.

The consumption of sugar is on the rise for many years and, despite the several warnings against these saturated fats, it is undoubtedly the greatest causative factor to high rate of diabetes epidemic.

Sugar consumption causes a number of physiological effects within the body. The most striking of these is the sudden increase in blood insulin which takes the food in our gut that has been broken down to the numerous sections of our body that require it.

First, and foremost importantly, glucose is very poisonous. If glucose is present in our bloodstream without control, increased levels of glucose would finish us quickly, so insulin release helps keep our blood safe and cleared of any excess glucose present in the body.

With our growing sedentary lifestyles needing to burn off much of the sudden and quick release of carbohydrate as we eat, sugar is rapidly converted to the exact same saturated fats we are constantly cautioned. (As you can see, restricting saturated fat from the diet doesn't stop us from accumulating fat in our bodies).

Sugar has other dangerous side effects. The constantly elevated insulin levels may finally lead to decreased insulin sensitivity and another instance of Type II diabetes. Sugar also competes with the glucose carriers in our blood, which operate with vitamins disrupts our immune system and causing premature skin aging.

Sugar is considered as nitro-fuel for the body. It releases a very quick burst of artificial energy. In busy people requiring peak performance from athletes, simple carbohydrates can be a useful tool, in the area of pre and post workout drinks.

Unfortunately few people utilize sugar in this cautious and controlled fashion and are trying to push the finely balanced engines of our bodies on a fuel which causes too much stress and strain on a method which was not designed to handle the excess we provide. So since low-carb diets nearly completely eliminate sugar from our diets, we have already found one important health advantage.

Ketoacidosis And Type 1 Diabetes

Ketoacidosis is something which is most likely to affect people with Type 1 Diabetes. This is a very severe diabetes complication that is caused by very substantial levels of acidity in blood.

The prefix - keto - is in reference to ketones, which are substances that your body creates as fat breaks during ketoacidosis. The expression acid a part of the title since the blood becomes acidic due to the presence of ketones.

There are some scenarios where Ketoacidosis is responsible for somebody discovering that they have type 1 diabetes. But it's much more common to happen after you've already discovered that you have the disease. Ketoacidosis ,mostly occurs in folks with type 1 diabetes, and most especially individuals who are over 40 year of age.

The main reason ketoacidosis occurs in individualswith type 1 diabetes is because their bodies don't have any natural insulin, it's just available when they inject it.

Those who have type 2 diabetes don't normally get ketoacidosis only because they do have insulin in their bodies, although it is not fully active on account of their body's immunity.

When people with type 2 diabetes do get ketoacidosis they do so when they've experienced a severe infection or have experience trauma that has put their own body under a great deal of stress.

The two most common causes of Ketoacidosis are an interruption of insulin treatment and infections. Those with type 1 diabetes are not able to really go for any hours on end without insulin until fat begins to be burnt for energy and begins to make extra sugar that the body cannot utilize. While this occurs, the burning fat creates ketones in your blood, which is responsible for ketoacidosis.

It's interesting to note that even if you don't have diabetes which you can be effected by a variant of this Condition if you go onto a really strict diet. Your body could very well begin to Burn some of its fat stores and produce ketones, just like it does in a diabetic.

The difference in this scenario is that while your blood glucose level stays low, you'll have sufficient insulin in your body to prevent an Excessive quantity of sugar to be generated, or using a sizable amount released By your liver.

Being on a rigorous diet normally does not lead to ketoacidosis, though your fat stores will probably be burned off. In someone without diabetes, this problem is known as ketosis and isn't dangerous.

The breakdown of body fat into tatty acids has as one of its side effects the formation of what is called ketones. These acidic by-products of fat metabolism possess the propensity of raising the body's acidity level when they accumulate in the bloodstream and may degenerate into specific health conditions.

One way by which ketones can accumulate in the blood is via the use of ketogenic diets. Ketogenic diets is of the opinion that carbohydrates are the significant cause of weight reduction and are so designed to limit the amount of carbs consumed daily in their own diets.

Carbohydrates are generally digested to produce glucose, which is considered to be the preferred energy source for the body. Although the body is capable of metabolizing muscle and liver glycogen (a combination of sugar and water) and body fat deposits to produce energy, it prefers to receive it from high glycemic index carbohydrates.

The initial phase of a ketogenic diet usually involves an acute deprivation of sugar designed to force the body to exhaust its available glucose to a considerably reduced level that finally compels it to change to burning its fat deposits for energy.

At this stage of a ketogenic diet, the rate of lipolysis (break down of body fat) increases radically to push the body into a condition known as ketosis in order to meet its energy requirements.

Ketosis is a state or condition in which the rate of formation of ketone bodies (by-products of this breakdown of fat into fatty acids) is faster than the rate at which they are being oxidized by body cells.

Ketone bodies are rapidly oxidized to water and carbon dioxide but also the increased accumulation in a state of ketosis creates their oxidation very hard.

However, the elevated accumulation of ketones in the blood generally leads to greater body acidity forcing the body to try using it water reservations out of its own cells to flush out the collected ketones.

Ketogenic diets are therefore designed to achieve two very important weight reduction goals that are: the decrease in insulin production on account of the resultant low blood sugar levels; and also the state of ketosis which increases the rate of lipolysis (fat break down). The combination of both of these factors makes the use of a ketogenic diet an extremely effective way of attaining rapid weight loss.

Regrettably, there has been some mix up regarding the state of increased ketone accumulation within the body. This is partially because of the simple fact that a lot of people fail to realize that besides the ketosis impact of ketogenic diets, another physiological condition may equally cause greater ketone accumulation.

Besides ketosis, ketoacidosis is the other condition which could result in an increased ketone accumulation. Even though there's absolutely no doubt that both conditions lead to greater accumulation of ketones and therefore acidity of the body, the precipitating conditions are however very different.

Diabetic Ketoacidosis - DKA is a serious condition whereby ketone bodies accumulate in the blood of Type I Diabetic men as a result of inability of the body to produce sufficient quantities of insulin. This problem is worsened by an increase in counter-regulatory hormones.

Insulin deficiency in a diabetic person contributes to hyperglycemia - an abnormal rise in blood glucose levels which can be as high as four times the normal quantity of sugar from the bloodstream.

In a normal individual, when there is an abnormal increase in blood sugar levels, glucose is filtered by the glomeruli and are reabsorbed by the kidney tubules, resulting in its excretion in the urine.

Hyperglycemia in and of itself is not that deadly but the side effects can be life threatening as it generally results in glycosuria (presence of sugar in the urine), dehydration, and increased urination. The loss of glucose in the urine normally leads to weakness, fatigue, weight loss, and increased appetite.

The continuing excretion of glucose in the pee along with the dehydration helps the entire body to become seriously starved of energy. To bring the problem under control, the human body may on the 1 hand continue excreting sugar in the urine resulting in a more severe condition,

Hyperosmolar Hyperglycemia Condition (HHS) - which has a proven mortality rate of about 15% in people with this condition.

On the other hand, the body may begin breaking down more triglycerides (stored body fat) as a means to make more energy to control the situation.

But this greater lipolysis (discharge of fatty acids and ketones from fat cells, muscle tissues and the liver) causes an elevated accumulation of ketones (the by-products of fat break down) in the urine and blood raising the acidity of the blood vessels The combination of both hyperglycemia and acidosis (abnormal increase in blood acidity) is what is known as Diabetic Ketoacidosis.

Therefore, while there is really an elevated amount of gathered ketones in both states, there's however increased blood glucose level in the state of ketoacidosis. Ketoacidosis can really clot to hyperventilation causing following impairment of central nervous system functions which can result in coma and death.

It has to be highlighted therefore, that dieters using ketogenic diets will need to ensure that they consume a good deal of water so as to decrease the higher acidity level of the body caused by the ketone accumulation. This also helps to flush out the collected ketones and to keep a condition of proper hydration.

While ketosis is due to low glucose levels, ketoacidosis is however brought on by increase glucose levels. Although ketone accumulation in the bloodstream and urine may be present in the two states, their causes are nevertheless poles apart.

Chapter 16
Keto For Lowering Convulsions

The ketogenic diet originates from the observation that fasting lowers convulsions. The brain usually uses only glucose as an energy source. However, carbohydrates are limited and fat is used as energy source in the brain during a ketogenic diet.

The liver is capable of converting fatty acids to so-called ketone bodies. Ketones can pass through the blood-brain barrier and serve as fuel for the brain's energy. These ketone bodies are hypothesized to be anticonvulsant in nature and to assist regulate convulsions.

In four stages, a patient takes a typical Indian ketogenic diet. The first stage consists primarily of a full medical history which includes the patient's private data and his / her diet. Anthropometric measures are carried out and fundamental blood and urine tests are carried out.

The second phase, also known as the "washout" of carbohydrates, involves limiting the amount of carbohydrates, so that the body moves from glucous to ketones. The diet omits all cereals, pulses, dhals, fruit and fruit juices, sucrum cane juice, cold beverages, sugar, jaggery, honey, sweets, chocolates, pudding and cakes.

Only elevated fat and protein foods are permitted. There is no quantity limitation. Once the body gets ketosis (the individual passes urine through ketones), the third stage begins.

The third stage includes maintaining ketosis using ketogenic ingredients. These are specific ingredients calculated by the ketogenic and nutritional unit amount (DUQ) ratios.

The fourth phase is then followed, which involves periodic follow-up with the doctor and nutritionist to allow fine tuning wherever necessary. The diet can be continued until seizures totally stop and the EEG normalizes.

The ketogenic diet is beneficial since it utilizes easy foods we eat every day. The price is nominal. Nothing must be imported and nothing is in risk of being inaccessible.

It's also a better option than neurochirurgy, which is very costly and includes both high risk. Naturally produced ketone bodies have anticonvulsant effects and fit without any side-effects. Medications can be reduced or omitted.

Patients on this diet were more alert with better concentration and memory. If a person is not satisfied with this diet, he must return to his original diet. There are, however, few side-effects related to the metabolic changes induced.

Hypoglycemia, dehydration, constipation, and vitamin or mineral deficiencies. Therefore, drinking plenty of water and taking multivitamin tablets on ketogenic diets is always advisable.

This diet emphasizes high fat, moderate protein, and low carbohydrates and is therefore definitely not developed for any weight loss as it is the opposite of any other diet you may think of.

Scientific studies, however, have shown that this diet can help reduce or prevent epilepsy in young people, even cases that can not be controlled by medication. It has been medically proven that over half of the youngsters on this diet have a 50% reduction in their seizures and at least 10-15% become seizure-free.

Most ketogenic diet children continue to take their seizure medicines but some can take smaller doses now that they are on this diet and depending on their physician this reduction can be started safely as early as this diet's initiation period.

Be very aware, however, that if the child goes off the diet[even for one meal] the effect of the diet may be lost, it is very difficult for the parent to get the child to maintain this diet at 100%, especially if the siblings eat normal diets and have free access to the fridge.

Strict youth control is needed and a dietitian could help design an interesting ketogenic diet that contains some of the child's favorite foods.

Meal example

Breakfast: cheese omelet, olive oil and steamed broccoli

Snack: cheese wedge

Lunch: hamburger patty with cheese and mayonnaise salad

Snack: protein shake with coconut oil

Dinner: salmon with asparagus and olive oil

This ketogenic diet forces the body into burning fats rather than carbohydrates[similar to the Atkins diet] and this generates glucose that we know helps.

This is due to the low intake of carbohydrate that forces the liver to convert fats into ketones, and as more ketones are produced the body becomes ketosis, this is beneficial for children with difficulty treating epilepsy as ketosis acts as an anti-convulsive.

1) Nausea and vomiting due to high-fat content can be minimized or prevented by a slow increase in fat over a few days.

2) Drowsiness and lethargy due to the increase in ketone levels, take note of the energy levels of the child before the diet and as your child adjusts to ketones, you will see an improvement in their alertness and much less drowsiness.

3) Constipation, a common side effect that can be avoided by good fluid intake, including high-fiber, low-carbon vegetables. Also, a daily dose of a stool softener could help the child with no ill effect.

4) Kidney stones are less common side effects, avoid this by ensuring a good daily fluid intake.

Chapter 17
Aerobic Exercise And
Ketogenic Weight Loss Plan

Aerobic exercise and ketogenic weight loss plan is the ideal combo you can encounter since most of us wishes to have a healthy and fit body. With 2 factors you can accomplish the body that you like but still, have sufficient energy to and so some exercise.

Diet will regularly be useless if you won't do a workout. Picture yourself losing weight but not having a firm and healthy physique. This is what'll happen to you if you lack a workout when having the diet. You might reduce weight but the body structure won't be in the shape that is perfect.

You will find firms that promote effective fat reduction solutions in addition to applications. That can purchase the best one you have to compare all these and know the difference.

You can set factors you will follow base from what you would like in a dietary program or product. With this process, it will get easier to determine what brand to purchase.

Ketogenic diet benefits are great for anybody who'll put it to use. With all the combination of cardio exercise and the ketogenic diet, you can be sure to be happy with the end result though you'll additionally be satisfied with it.

A lot of things happens when you are working out. Several of these are great for the health and some aren't so great - like if you exercise excessively.

Physical exercise is a stressor. Although it can be an excellent stressor, it will, however, trigger the adrenals going into overdrive. This situation increases the insulin levels and thus reduces the ability to slim down.

When working out, the insulin levels go up while the hunger reduces. Nevertheless, this often leads to a considerable decrease in blood glucose levels which results for you becoming hungrier. It is crucial that you note that actually, a reasonable rise in insulin levels causes a tremendous lowering of lipolysis or fat loss.

One issue we have when we wish to slim down is we concentrate a lot on the figures showing on the machine. We almost unconsciously overlook probably the most crucial thing which is losing excess fat.

We have more than eighty % of the body fat stored in body fat cells. To be equipped to eliminate this stored extra fat, one would have to burn it for energy generation. Nevertheless, before the body can start burning your stored weight for energy, there is the need to have a bad fat balance.

If the body is now used to losing fat for energy, it can today use both body fat and dietary fat for energy. This is among the primary key energy of utilizing a ketogenic diet for slimming down.

When you don't increase the dietary fat intake but raise the quantity of energy the body requires through increasing the exercise intensity, your body is going to get just about all of that energy from burning excess fat.

Nevertheless, in case the body is fueled with carbohydrates, you'll mainly be burning sugar for energy. This will make it a lot hard for the body to burn and lose excess fat. It is however vital that you understand that while exercise can enable you to slim down, it is essential to get the diet properly initially.

When you have the correct diet, by making use of a ketogenic diet, the body will begin making use of the fat deposits for producing the energy which effectively allows you to start burning & losing excess fat.

Once the body is used to the ketogenic diet, you'll feel more energetic. At such a place, you will be better positioned to adjust the menus that can begin building muscles and strength.

If you reach this time throughout the "standard ketogenic" diet, you can then modify the diet plan to possibly a "targeted" or a "cyclical" ketogenic diet plan. These types of the ketogenic diet enable more carbohydrate consumption to allow you to indulge in more workouts for longer.

Specific Ketogenic Diet

The Targeted Ketogenic Diet enables you to ingest a lot of carbs around the exercise period. This type of diet enables you to participate with high-intensity exercise while currently staying in ketosis.

The carb intake inside this window offers the muscles together with the required glucose to properly engage in the workouts. The additional glucose should usually be used up during this particular window of approximately thirty minutes and shouldn't affect the overall metabolism.

The Targeted Ketogenic Diet is created for newbies or intermittent exercisers. The TKD enables a slight rise in carb consumption. Nevertheless, it doesn't kick you out there ketosis and leads to no shock to the system.

Cyclical Ketogenic Diet

The Cyclical Ketogenic Diet is more adequate for advanced bodybuilders and athletes. It is frequently used for optimum muscle-building results.

There is however an energy full tendency for others to wind up introducing several excess fats. This is since it is so easy to overindulge while utilizing the Cyclical Ketogenic Diet (CKD).

In this particular edition of the ketogenic diet plan, the person uses the conventional ketogenic diet for five or six days. He or she is therefore permitted to consume increased quantities of carbohydrate for one or two days.

As a care, it can have a novice close to three months to completely get back to ketosis when he or she tries the CKD. It takes real commitment and experienced physical amounts to effectively do a CKD.

The target of the Cyclical Ketogenic Diet would be to temporarily transition of ketosis. This particular window provides the body the chance to refill the quantity of glycogen in the muscles to allow it to tackle the following cycle of workouts that are intense.

Thus, there has to be a total depletion of the resulting glycogen build up throughout the subsequent routines that can get back to ketosis. The intensity of your respective planned workout will consequently figure out the quantity of increased carb consumption.

If you exercise at a rigorous rate, a lot of things that are amazing happen to the body.

If you indulge in aerobic exercises, they help you to enhance the effectiveness of your lungs and heart. This additionally helps to boost the rate at which the body burns energy and over time this can result in loss of weight.

Engaging with cardio exercise leads to numerous metabolic modifications which positively affect fat metabolic rate. Cardiovascular exercises help to boost oxygen delivery through improved blood circulation. This particular manner, body cells are in a position to better oxidize and melt fat.

This has got the outcome of boosting the variety of oxidative enzymes. So, the pace at what fatty acids are moved to the mitochondria to be used for energy is significantly improved.

Throughout cardio exercises, the sensitivity of fat cells and muscles to epinephrine is significantly improved. This increases the number of triglycerides which are introduced into the blood and muscles to be used for energy.

Toughness Training

Strength training helps to enhance the moods while simultaneously helping to build wholesome bones. Additionally, it allows you to develop a generally strong and body that is healthy.

With a well-designed ketogenic plan is going to help you preserve the muscles while carrying the strength training. Muscles are designed with protein, not fat loss or carbs.

Additionally, because of the simple fact that protein oxidation is less money in a ketogenic diet, partaking with strength training shouldn't be an issue. You have to challenge the body with heavy weights to actually see results and also get a better body.

Interval Training

Interval training is just alternating intervals of high-intensity and low-intensity workouts. It is merely for you to: go fast, go slow, and do this.

While sounding quite simple, interval training is but one of the most effective methods to burn excess fat fast. Apart from burning body fat while holding away interval training, the "afterburn effect" induces the metabolism for an extended time period.

Circuit Training: Cardio + Strength Circuit training is essentially the merging of aerobic workouts with strength training workouts. This combination helps to offer all over fitness benefits.The absence of sleep in between equal exercises earn circuit training as helpful as a cardio-based high-intensity interval training workout.

Chapter 18
Ketogenic Diet For Bipolar Patients

Ketone bodies are three different biochemicals produced as by-products when fatty acids break down for energy. Two of the three are the brain's energy source.

Neurotransmitters (such as serotonin and dopamine) work by varying these membrane potentials. Neurotransmitters has the ability to open ion channels, thus allowing sodium to enter into the cell, causing an electrical impulse wave that travels in the path of the neuron.

That's the problem in bipolar patients, especially serotonin and dopamine neurotransmitters. The synapse region does not allow a message from one neuron to pass correctly to another neuron, making one react inappropriately to a situation, sometimes with little inhibition.

When a person is in a ketogenic state, sodium mediation opens the electrical impulses that pass from neuron to neuron. It allows extracellular calcium to pour into the cell, leading to release serotonin and dopamine neurotransmitters into the synapse region.

Then, depending on the situation, it can be released to the next neuron to generate a suitable response, like excitement or inhibition.

The ketogenic diet and macronutrients are protein, fat, and carbohydrates. Ketogenic diets limit carbohydrate intake to 20 grams or less per day. Each gram has four calories, each gram has four calories, and each gram has nine calories.

This results in most of your caloric intake from proteins and fat. Ketone bodies are made of fat, which your brain uses as fuel instead of carbohydrate glucose. Acetoacetate and beta-hydroxybutyrate are acidic.

Protons can be pumped into neurons in exchange for sodium, acting like lithium, a common drug prescribed for bipolar patients. Extra protons outside the cell help do things like decrease neuron excitability and decrease serotonin and dopamine neurotransmitter excitatory activity.

Ketogenic Diet Limitations for Bipolar Patients

Several studies by people using ketogenic diet plans to improve their bipolar symptoms can be found online. Unfortunately, no scientific studies support the findings of using a ketogenic diet to treat bipolar patients.

As you would find in bipolar patients, a ketogenic diet similar to the one used for epilepsy has stabilizing and antidepressant effects. And the Standford Medical School tried studying bipolar patients using a ketogenic diet protocol. Unfortunately, the trial never began due to the inability to attract subjects. But, this proves they felt a study warranted.

Another limitation is the dietary carbohydrate restriction. If one is limited to 20 or fewer grams of carbohydrates per day, they must select low-glycemic index-scale vegetables. The glycemic index is a numerical scale used to calculate how fast food raises blood sugar.

Like broccoli, spinach, and iceberg lettuce, which only contain one or two carbohydrates per cup, foods low on GI must be incorporated. And to avoid all complex carbohydrates like grains, pasta, and bread.

Just one slice of bread can have 20 grams of carbs. This can make staying on the diet a difficult task given the limited amount of carbohydrates allowed, limiting food choices.

While scientific evidence lagged in showing empirical findings that a ketonic diet works well for bipolar patients, there was sufficient evidence that it is gaining attention, as at the Standford Medical School. And scientific evidence shows that it does similar things to brain neurotransmitters as does lithium, a common bipolar patient medication.

Chapter 19
Ketogenic Dieting For
Treating Migraines

ketogenic diet helps squash migraines ketones happen. A ketogenic diet relates to one low in carbohydrates, enabling the body to break down fat to metabolize ketones quicker.

Foods allow the body to create ketones are MCT oil known as medium-chain triglycerides, Grass-fed butter and coconut oil The significant factor about ketones is that they help you get rid of migraines.

Here are the top 7 ways ketones squash migraines:

1: reduced migraine frequency Recent trials have discovered that the ketogenic diet considerably lowered migraine frequency in 90% of patients. This dwarfs the impacts of migraine.

2: Glutamate inhibition Epilepsy and migraine find glutamate. Epileptic (anti-seizure) medications also block glutamate production. These drugs also used to treat migraines. Since about 500 BC, ketones have worked to avoid seizures, but ketogenic diet has only been common for the last century.

3: Processed food I've repeatedly said that processed foods are bad for you, particularly if you have migraine. "Food-like goods" contain preservatives, chemicals, and other causes that may influence your symptoms. Any diet removing processed foods, including ketogenic diet, would be a nice move to manage migraine symptoms.

4: Saturated fats Several trials revealed a fat myth. A ketogenic diet includes plenty of saturated fats (and other healthy fats) that have been discovered to decrease bad cholesterol and help the body generate serotonin and vitamin D, both helping prevent migraines.

5: Hunger vs. weight management Hunger is a significant trigger and weight gain / obesity. Some trials discovered that weight gain and/or obesity increased migraine risk by 81%. Ketones assist decrease hunger by managing insulin issues, encouraging weight loss, and regulating blood glucose.

Weight loss and sugar control are known to add MCT or coconut oil to your diet. As you can see, they will assist manage migraines by helping you feel nutritionally happy, more energetic, enhance cognitive functioning, and lose fat.

6: Oxidative stress Recent research discovered migraine-related oxidative stress. Following these results, a fresh migraine medication appeared blocking the peptide released during oxidative stress.

It also avoids glutamate, another migraine cause. You don't need medication, though. A ketogenic diet will do both for you, suggesting that ketones can treat migraine symptoms as well as recognize the root cause.

7: MCT Oil Research discovered patients with Alzheimer's response to MCT oil, particularly memory recall. Migraine patients do have white-matter brain lesions. Research has discovered that ketones can help boost brain metabolism even when oxidative stress and glucose intolerance happen.

Our minds and bodies need oxygen and/or ketones. We store about 24 hours of sugar in our bodies, but if not ketones, we'd all die of hypoglycemia. Metabolizing fat ketones leaves us in good ketosis.

Migraines indicate that the brain doesn't correctly metabolize glucose into energy, so adding ketones is the logical reaction. A ketogenic diet can also assist: block glutamate (a significant trigger) Eliminate processed foods (a significant trigger)

Chapter 20
Sugar, Fat And Protein Precaution On The Ketogenic Diet

Keto shifts the body from a high sugar burner to a fat burner by reducing the nutritional sugars produced from carbs. The very first apparent reduction you need to make from the current diet is sugary foods and sugar.

We need to look out for sugar in a variety of various types of nutrients and foods. Actually, a white potato might not be sweet to the tongue like sugar. But the moment it hits the bloodstream following digestion, those carbs include the easy sugar known as sugar to the body.

The fact is, the body will only keep a lot of sugar before it dumps it somewhere else in the system. Excessive glucose becomes what is referred to as the weight which accumulates in the stomach region, love handles, etcetera.

Proteins And It is Place In Keto

One source of carbs which many people overlook in the diet is protein. Overconsumption of protein-based on the tolerance amount of the body is going to result in fat gain.

Since the body converts unwanted protein to sugar, we should moderate the quantity of protein we consume. The protein intake is an element of how you can eat ketogenic and lose pounds.

To begin with, determine your own tolerance of regular use and protein as a guide to keep an ideal consumption of the nutrient. Next, choose the protein from foods like organic eggs and meats. Lastly, create food in variety which is scrumptious and maintains the interest in the diet plan.

The Ketogenic Diet Caloric Intake

Calories are another vital consideration for what are you can consume on a ketogenic diet plan. The energy produced from the calories in the meals we consume assist the body to stay functional. Hence, we should eat sufficient calories in order to satisfy the daily nutritional requirements.

Calorie counting is a burden for a lot of people who are on some other diets. But as a ketogenic dieter, you do not need to be concerned almost so much about calorie counting. Many people on a low carb diet plan stay happy by consuming an everyday amount of 1500 1700 kcals in calories.

Fat, The Good & The Bad

Fat isn't bad, actually, some excellent wholesome oils occur in whole foods like nuts, olive oil, and seeds.

Fats that are healthy are a fundamental component of the ketogenic diet regime and can be found as spreads, toppings, and snacks. Misconceptions with respect to consuming body fat are that a high quantity of it is bad and leads to fat gain.

While both claims are located in a sense correct, the weight that we ingest isn't the immediate cause of the fat that shows up in the body. Instead, the sugar out of each nutrient we consume is exactly what ultimately turns into the fat on the body.

Balance The Nutrients

Digestion will cause sugars we consume to take in into the bloodstream and the extra length transfer in the fat cells. High carbohydrate and protein eating can result in extra body fat because there is sugar in these nutrients.

Therefore substantial eating of any substance is bad and leads to fat gain. Though a nutritious diet plan is composed of a balance of proteins, carbs & oils based on the tolerance amounts of the body.

Nearly everyone can accomplish a ketogenic diet with sufficient effort and persistence. Additionally, we can moderate a selection of bodily conditions obviously with keto. Insulin resistance, elevated blood glucose, obesity, inflammation, type 2 diabetes are a few health issues which keto could help to stabilize.

All these bad conditions will lessen and normalize for the victim that follows a proper ketogenic diet plan. Low-carb, moderate and high-fat protein wholesome foods provide life-changing health advantages from this diet.

While on a ketogenic diet plan, it is really important to make sure that an individual consumes inside the limitations of the diet. This is essential and so as for the person to have the ability to stay in a state of ketosis.

Going out of ketosis is often as easy as eating one or 2 meals which are not advised on the diet. Nevertheless, coming back to ketosis is yet another different story entirely. This can frequently take days or weeks based on just how strict you get if you get back on the diet plan.

Ketogenic diet programs by nature involve the intake of increased amounts of fat in the diet. They are available as part of the baking process or as dressings and sauces.

The most effective kinds of oils are all those medium-chain triglycerides (MCTs). These consist of both MCT oil and coconut oil. Medium-chain triglycerides are very easily metabolized to create ketones.

When purchasing the protein foods, constantly attempt to choose grass-fed, natural and humanely raised meat and wild-caught seafood. Apart from providing far more nutrition, they haven't been subjected to added hormones, antibiotics, and any other likely toxins.

Meat

The ketogenic diet accepts essentially any meat type. There is no discrimination about the kind of preparation or cut.

Beef, Goat, Lamb, Pork, Veal, Venison

Poultry

Any kind of poultry is allowed by the diet plan. You can enhance the information in the meal by making the skin feed on it. Nevertheless, batter and breading shouldn't be utilized in the preparing of poultry as they are normally loaded with carbs. Besides that, you can prepare the poultry to your liking.

Chicken, Pheasant, Quail, Squab, Goose, Ostrich, Partridge, Duck, Game hen, Turkey

Seafood

Yet another excellent source of protein is seafood. Seafood is a terrific source of omega 3 essential fatty acids. Additionally, they have very high amounts of vitamins and minerals to help keep you healthy and well-nourished.

Clams, Oysters, Prawns, Scallops, Crab, Lobster, Mussels, Shrimp, Snails

Fish

Fish have many good amounts of omega-3 essential fatty acids. You will go for fish which are found in the outdoors and in mercury-free places.

Ahi, Tuna, Trout, Swordfish, Squid, Snapper, Scallops, Sardines, Salmon, Mussel, Mahi Mahi, Mackerel, Lobster, Herring, Halibut, Flounder, Cod, Catfish, Walleye

Carbohydrates

Vegetables

Veggies have become the main source of carbohydrate on a ketogenic diet plan. When you are purchasing vegetables usually choose natural organic vegetables. Furthermore, the dark leafy vegetables have a minimum amount of carbs with excellent nutrition.

Arugula, Swiss chard, Spinach, Seaweed, Radishes, Peppers, Onions, Mushrooms, Lettuce, Kelp, Kale, Garlic, Endive, Celery, Collard greens, Cauliflower, Cabbage, Broccoli, Bok choy, Asparagus, Watercress

Milk and Dairy products These are really important in a ketogenic diet plan. Organic and grass-fed supply tend to be more preferable. The total fat type is a bit better suited for the ketogenic diet regime compared to the low-fat and fat-free verities.

Butter, Cheddar, Crème fraîche, Heavy cream, Mozzarella, Sour cream, Cream cheese, Mascarpone cheese, Cheeses, Hard cheeses

Nuts

Reasonable quantities of nuts and seed are permitted on the ketogenic diet plan. Nuts and seed are loaded with protein, fat, and carbohydrates. The entire fat, carbohydrate and protein content of the nut variations should be examined and also added to the entire daily calorie calculation.

Nuts that are roasted and seeds are the very best. Something that could cause harm or even interfere with ketosis within the body has been removed from them throughout the roasting process.

Nuts should be utilized generally as a snack

Almonds, Macadamia, and Walnuts are several of the best

A number of nuts have a high content of omega 6 fatty acid that will bring about inflammation within the body. Nevertheless, they can store some individuals again from the goals. But if the weight loss is solely the purpose of utilizing the ketogenic diet, then simply it will be best to eliminate seeds and nuts to boost the results.

Almonds, Sunflower seeds, Sesame seeds, Pumpkin seeds, Pili nuts, Pecans, Macadamia nuts, Pine nuts, Hazelnuts, Brazil nuts, Walnuts

Spices and herbs After a while on the ketogenic diet plan, the meals might begin to be dull. To add spices to the meals may however assist to spice things up. You can add dry and fresh spices to the meals and beverages so that they be more enticing and enjoyable to the palate.

Fresh herbs and spices are several of the most nutrient-dense foods in the world you can eat. Adding spices to the meal does not just increase the flavors to the meals but additionally offer a lot of various health advantages to the body.

Spices contain carbohydrates hence you need to ensure to put them to the daily carbohydrate count. Additionally, endeavor to look at the labeling of built-in spice mixes for the accurate carbohydrate content because they typically contain added sugars.

Salt additionally improves flavors. It is best you chose good quality sea salt rather than regular table salt. Unprocessed salts, for instance, Celtic or Himalayan sea salt offers you over 8 trace minerals your body need to function well.

Anise, Turmeric, Thyme, Tarragon, Star anise, Spearmint, Sage, Saffron, Rosemary, Peppermint, Parsley, Paprika, Oregano, Mustard seeds, Mint, Marjoram, Mace, Licorice, Lemongrass, Ginger, Garlic, Galangal, Fenugreek, Dill, Curry, Cumin, Coriander, Cloves, Cinnamon, Cilantro, Chives, Chili pepper, Chervil, Celery seed, Cayenne pepper, Caraway Cardamom, Black pepper, Bay leaf, Basil, Annatto, Vanilla beans

Sweeteners

Adding artificial sweeteners to the meals can assist in curbing cravings for sweets and carbohydrates. Sweeteners help a large number of individuals to have the ability to stick to the ketogenic diet.

Nevertheless, natural sweeteners for example honey, maple syrup, and agave raise blood glucose levels which don't just result in inflammation but also can kick you of ketosis.

Constantly aim for the liquid form of sweeteners as they don't have binders as maltodextrin and dextrose. Dextrose is an anti-caking agent and it is a kind of sugar. Maltodextrin on the flip side is a bulking representative that has a higher glycemic index (110) than table sugar (fifty-two).

The following is a summary of suggested sweeteners which happen to have little impact on blood glucose.

Blended sweeteners (Sukrin, Swerve, Lakanto), Erythritol, Stevia, Monk Fruit, Stevia glycerite (a heavy liquid form of stevia), Xylitol, Sucralose.

Beverages

With a low carbohydrate diet just like the ketogenic diet plan has a diuretic impact on the entire body. Carbs draw water to them that result in water retention within the body. Nevertheless, the reduced carbohydrate ingestion in a ketogenic diet plan leads to a lot of water loss as less h2o is retained within the body and more is excreted.

This particular diuretic effect can readily lead to dehydration. So you have to consume a great deal of water - well above the suggested intake of eight cups - when you are on a ketogenic diet plan. This can enable you to lessen the danger of urinary tract and bladder pain infections.

Besides water, you can add other types of beverages like teas and coffee to help you maintain hydration during the day. Both of these don't substantially impact the ketosis state.

Nevertheless, the additional substances as milk and sugar could possibly influence the ketosis state. As an outcome, it will be better to stay away from the sugar completely and buy either artificial sweeteners or full cream together with your tea or coffee.

An alternate way to boost the beverage intake is making vegetable juice by blending sorts of the approved vegetable sorts. You can additionally make use of energy smoothies or protein shakes rather than a berry smoothies as the fruits have sugars (fructose) which could kick you of ketosis.

Below are a few extra drinks you can take in to keep you hydrated: Unsweetened milk, money milk, coconut milk, hemp milk, Green tea extract, Organic caffè Americano, Mineral water.

Chapter 21
What Foods To Avoid On The Keto Diet?

Because you're going to focus on fat and protein— and go easy on carbs— big pasta bowls (or any grain, really) definitely won't be on your menu. It also means that starchy vegetables like potatoes and carrots and legumes like chickpeas, lentils, and black beans are also off-limits.

Something else you can't have: sweets—natural or artificial. Cakes, candy, and doughnuts are a no; and many fruits (apples, bananas, pears— all have tons of sugar, which is definitely a carb) are not allowed.

Another gray area on the keto diet— many sugary cocktails and beers are banned on the keto diet, along with some sweeter wines.

Note: Since you are excluding some major keto diet food groups (grains, many fruits), you should definitely consider taking a multivitamin— especially one that contains folic acid that helps your body make new cells and is often found in enriched breads, cereals, and other grain products.

Does the keto diet have side-effects?

It usually takes your body three to four days to go into ketosis because you must first use glucose stores in your body, i.e. sugar. Any major diet change can give you problems, uh.

These issues can be part of what's called "keto flu," Warren says. Other side effects of the keto diet may include nausea, mental fog, cramps, lightheadedness, and headaches, as well as tiredness. Luckily, keto flu usually doesn't last more than a week— which is coincidentally about when people start seeing the number dropping on the scale.

Besides typical keto flu complaints, keto breath and diarrhea are also common keto side effects.

While diarrhea may be another symptom of keto flu, it could be linked to how your body processes fat, (and, as you know, fat-filled keto diet). The reason: some people just don't digest fat as they should.

On the other hand, keto breath is less of a side-effect and more of a harmless inconvenience (your breath literally smells like nail polish remover). When your body breaks down all that extra fat on the keto diet, it generates ketones— one of which is chemical acetone.

Your body is then destroyed by defecation, urination,and, breathing. Keto breath should disappear once your body's diet acclimates— meanwhile, pay special attention to your oral hygiene.

Okay, I'm dying to know: will the diet help me lose weight?

As mentioned, there are a few reasons why keto diet usually equals gold weight-loss. For starters, people usually reduce their daily caloric intake to about 1,500 calories a day because healthy fats and lean proteins make you feel fuller earlier— and longer.

There is the fact that processing and burning protein and fats require more energy than carbs, so you will be burning more calories than before. Over time, this can cause weight loss.

Everyone is unique, and how much you weigh when you begin your diet matters, but on keto, you could safely lose about 1-2 pounds a week. "It's sometimes more or less, depending on the caloric needs of the individual. Keto diet is not a" miracle meat burner.

"Fat calories are still calories, so working out and maintaining full consumption in a sensitive way is the only way to work." You can still add fat to the frame if you are on keto diet but eat more calories than you need.

Many people testify that intermittent fasting is great for weight loss, but any results you would see are short-lived. In other words, if you start eating regularly, you gain weight back.

"Combining a restrictive diet with long non-eating is non-ideal. "The body cannibalizes its own muscle for energy if food intake is too low, but the body doesn't distinguish between something like a calf muscle or heart muscle.

Keep in mind that all your significant organs are made up of smooth muscle, and being on a diet like this can damage your lungs or bladder like fat loss. "Science on IF so far has been quite evident that weight loss from intermittent fasting is due to calorie restriction. And, a study has shown, eating less, or healthier overall generally does the same thing.

You literally starve to a fasting diet. Methods like this are appealing because weight loss can vary from 1-4 pounds a week, but mainly the lean muscle is essential for the healthy functioning as you age, and it is very difficult to recover once the muscle has been gone.

Trying this is not recommended if you do not have it with your doctor or nutritionist to make sure it fits you and your lifestyle.

When something is popular, it ensures that people find new or easier ways of doing it. Enter the dirty, lazy diets of keto. With lazy keto, people try to limit their carbohydrate to 20 to 50 grams a day, but don't really track it; with dirty keto, they typically have the same macronutrient breakdown as regular keto, but wherever they come from doesn't matter.

Chapter 22
Changing Your Food Environment

Being out of the safe prepared environment of a keto-friendly home can be a real challenge, but it doesn't have to be as daunting as it may seem.

A few easy modifications can discourage weight gain while traveling: carry keto-friendly snacks. Having food readily on hand will reduce the likelihood of just grabbing anything you can get your hands on, maintaining your cravings at bay, and avoiding overeating.

Do your studies before leaving.

If you know where you're going, visit menus and accessible shops to discover particular keto-friendly alternatives.

Don't beat a slight deviation.

If you're away for a few days, it won't hurt reaching out for some local food. While traveling, you don't have to remain on keto for weight loss and weight gain. As long as your choices are sensible and active, a short deviation won't throw you off track.

Introduce MCT Oil

Research shows that the advantages of medium-chain triglycerides (MCTs), also known as' friendly fat,' are great to support the body to guarantee outstanding dietitian outcomes.

MCT's are digested in different way from other fats as they reach the liver where they become ketones.

Elevated ketones assist your body achieve ketosis quicker, and many reported enhanced cognitive energy and feeling less hungry. Other beneficial advantages include enhanced well-being and thermogenic impacts to quicker fat burning.

Experts indicate that MCT oil is more efficient than coconut oil because it includes fewer fat-chain carbons that are absorbed quicker into the body.

Adding exogenous ketone salts as dietary health supplements is an efficient way to assist raise blood ketone concentrations more than is generally feasible with diet alone.

Top-quality exogenous ketones assist support the body during the keto diet in a number of ways, including: speeding up ketosis

Maintaining ketosis

Staying off keto flu

Restoring missed electrolytes

Suppressing appetite Increasing power

A quality exogenous supplement must contain at least 3 to 4 kinds of BHB derived ketone salts, such as calcium, sodium, and potassium. If you discover an MCT oil supplement, you're a winner. Effective daily serving should average 2000 mg.

4Be active and practice the first few weeks on keto is not a nice time to attempt a fresh workout, so remember when you begin. Once keto flu's initial symptoms have subsided (which can occur in the first few weeks), it's time to add exercise and activity to the mix.

General recommendation involves continuing your usual routines, but not introducing anything fresh until ketosis and keto flu have passed.

Fuel Your Body

Keto dieters tend to undereat as they exclude an entire carbs owed to the fact that the keto diet suppresses appetite so that the body may not obtain sufficient power to operate efficiently.

Reducing calories and exercise routine will likely make you feel unwell and affect your performance. Check what you eat before working out, and make sure you consume enough fat calories.

Choose Exercise Type Wisely You may need to rethink your exercise routine, and what once worked for you may no longer suit your keto.

Although diets high in a specific macronutrient such as fat produce an enhanced capacity to use that macronutrient as fuel, the body utilizes glycogen as fuel regardless of macronutrient consumption during high-intensity workouts (such as HIIT and CrossFit).

Glycogen stores are carb-fuelled, so if you don't consume them in large quantities, high-intensity exercise outcomes can be adversely impacted. Alternatively, moderate-intensity exercises are more suitable to increase the body's fat-burning potential.

Consider Intermittent Fasting Keto as the ultimate combo for weight shedding and wellness optimization.

Intermittent fasting is a window of hours when you can eat. You can do several forms, but the end outcome is the same, it helps control calorie and regulate insulin production. The approach chosen will determine your objectives and lifestyle.

The most common IF techniques are: time-limited eating-(e.g. 16/8 or 14/10) where you can eat 8 or 10 hours a day and the remainder of the time quickly.

Bi-weekly 5:2-twice weekly, restricted to 500 calories.

Similar to the 5:2 calorie limit strategy, but every other day.

Fasting-involves a full-day quickly. Usually once or twice daily.

The advantages mentioned include enhanced gut health, giving your digestive system a welcome break from the most prevalent eating / snacking pattern.

Intermittent fasting was strongly related to enhanced weight loss

Cognitive function and Boosted energy

Reduced insulin resistance & helps avoid diabetes Lowered LDL (poor cholesterol) Increased longevity

Chapter 23
The Unwanted Side Effects Of Using A Ketogenic Diet For Weight Loss

Ketogenic diet programs are created to make the body enter into a state called ketosis. The human body typically uses carbohydrate as the primary source of energy. This owes to the point that carbs would be the least difficult for the body to take in.

Nevertheless, when the body operates from carbohydrates, it reverts to making use of protein and fats for energy production.

Ketosis efficiently alters your body 's natural equation from burning up glucose to rather begin losing fat as fuel. This particular modification of the body 's metabolic process can come with a few potential unwanted side effects as the body attempts to regulate its functioning.

Changing to the ketogenic diet plan isn't that simple to adjust to particularly at the original onset. Nevertheless, keep in mind that these unwanted side effects are temporary. Several of them last for a couple of days while some other last for months.

So you have to provide yourself time, both mentally and physically, to successfully create the switch.

While making the switch to a ketogenic diet plan, you will find 2 actual physical changes that you might experience. These are the keto flu and keto breath.

Keto Flu

This is 1 thing that anybody starting a ketogenic diet must brace up for. It is an ailment that you have several of the various side effects which come together with using a ketogenic diet plan.

Keto flu is usually characterized by lightheadedness or even mind fogginess, stomachaches, nausea, headaches, and muscle soreness. You might additionally experience heightened feelings of lethargy, irritability and difficulty concentrating.

Interestingly, these are almost all typical signs of the flu, thus the name. These indicators are temporary and not everybody utilizing a ketogenic is impacted by them.

These indicators are usually brought on by the high sugar withdrawal occasioned by the substantially decreased carb consumption. Additionally, an imbalance in the body electrolytes for example calcium, potassium, magnesium, and salt can impact the way your body responds to the outcome of a ketogenic diet plan.

Keto Breath

You will find 2 possible explanations put forth exactly why folks on ketogenic diets encounter this unusual breath issue.

The human body doesn't save ketones and therefore they have to be excreted through the body. Ketones will be excreted from the urine as acetoacetate.

They could additionally be excreted from the breath in the type of acetone. And so the more ketones you create, the more acetone you pass out through the breath. Regrettably, this could cause unpleasant smelling breath when utilizing a ketogenic diet.

On the flip side, increased protein ingestion could additionally cause keto breath. This is since the manner the body digest fats and proteins are pretty different. The digestion of proteins frequently produces ammonia that the body excretes throughout the urine.

Nevertheless, the increased intake of proteins might lead to the indigestible amounts staying in the gut system and undergoes fermentation. This generates ammonia that is subsequently released through the breath.

Keto breath can keep going for about a week to under a month. It mainly depends on how nicely the body adapts to ketosis.

Micronutrient Deficiencies

This might end up from the rigid restrictions on carbohydrate consumption. A lot of carbohydrate-rich foods are equally abundant in minerals and vitamins.

The serious restriction on carbohydrate intake might thus cause deficiencies in certain important nutrients. Consequently, we shouldn't merely be centered on the micronutrient counting in the terminology of carbohydrates, proteins, and fat but must also recall the vitamin and mineral micronutrient contents also.

This is oftentimes why supplements are mainly recommended when utilizing a ketogenic diet. Supplementation is going to help to augment virtually any micronutrient imbalance that might happen when utilizing a ketogenic diet plan. Using a weight reduction diet just like the ketogenic diet can truly enable you to fast-track the weight loss efforts.

Chapter 24
What's The Proof That
Ketogenic Diet Works?

A ketogenic diet is relatively small in protein (eating more meat, eggs, chicken, fish, cheese or tofu) and low in fat, with recommended olive oil, coconut oil, nuts and seeds, and high-fat dairy foods such as cheese and butter.

It also allows fruit and vegetables like cabbage, berries, avocado, leafy greens, mushrooms, and citrus fruits.

Sample day: breakfast: two olive-fried eggs, sautéed spinach and tomato morning tea: a handful of nuts Lunch: chicken stir-fry with cauliflower sauce.

A cup of strawberries Dinner: steak with greens cooked in olive oil Why?

Initially, the ketogenic diet was created in the 1920s as epilepsy medical therapy (more on this below), but in popular culture it is now filtering through as a selection of celebrity-endorsed health and lifestyle.

Diet advocates point to weight loss and maintenance as just some of the benefits of a ketogenic diet.

Following ketogenic diet significantly increases protein and fat consumption.

What's the proof?

Promising study promotes ketogenic diet as a medical therapy for childhood epilepsy instances. While it is not understood exactly how it works, studies have shown that a ketogenic diet can help reduce seizures in drug-free children. Most research, however, is limited to small, child-only studies, so cannot be applied to the entire population.

Some studies among overweight and obese adolescents show that very low carbohydrate diets can be more effective in the short term (up to six months) than periodic, energy-restricted diets. But there's little to no long-term (up to five years) difference between the two approaches.

And when looking at risk factors for cardiovascular disease, some studies found both benefits and disadvantages to ketogenic diet; while some studies reported higher weight loss and improvements in HDL (or healthy cholesterol) followers either had less overall and improved LDL (or unhealthy cholesterol) or increased LDL cholesterol compared to low-fat diets.

Similar to research on epilepsy, researchers noted in long-term weight loss researches that followers found it hard to stick to, and also found that most carbohydrate intakes were not low enough to kick between 36-100 g daily.

So it's hard to draw conclusions about the suitability of the ketogenic diet for weight loss and long-term health compared to a low-carbohydrate diet.

Due to the fewer amount of carbohydrates allowed, a true ketogenic diet is difficult to follow—just 50 g daily.

Why can't I?

While burning fat sounds like an effective manner to lose weight, a long-term diet is tough. High drop-out rates and bad study compliance are partially why the ketogenic diet lacks research—because it's extremely restrictive, it's difficult to keep.

Ketosis implies that our body releases chemicals in breath, urine, and blood called ketones. This signals the body's fuel change and can result in significant, unpleasant side effects.

And due to its high fat content, it can cause side effects like constipation, abdominal cramps, diarrhea and vomiting, many consider the diet unpalatable and inconvenient for social situations.

By removing most carbohydrate-rich foods, sticking on ketosis implies missing a variety of healthy ingredients such as grains, fruit, vegetables, and legumes. Rich in fiber, minerals, vitamins, and phytochemicals, these foods can assist in protecting against chronic diseases such as colorectal cancer ,type 2 diabetes, and cardiovascular disease.

These foods also keep us satisfied between meals and help maintain good digestive systems as our gut feeds on resistant starch discovered in many carbohydrate-rich foods. Otherwise, our gut may not work at its best, and evidence to maintain diverse microbiota continues to grow, and the role of gut health in our overall health.

After a ketogenic diet, side effects like constipation, cramping, and vomiting aren't unusual.

What's the ultimate?

Ketogenic diets peak in popularity this year, but without strong evidence to support them, you don't need to feel pressured to cut off carbohydrate foods without medical advice. In fact, eating fruit, vegetables, grains and legumes as part of a balanced diet will boost your body with healthy foods to protect your health in the short and long term.

After about two to seven days after the keto diet, you're going into something called ketosis, or your body's state enters when your cells don't have enough energy carbs. When you begin producing ketones, or organic compounds, you use the missing carbs instead. Your body is now burning fat for more energy.

Believe it or not, keto diet was originally intended to help people with seizure disorders— not help people lose weight, says New York-based R.D. Jessica Cording. That's because ketones and other diet chemicals called decanoic acid can help minimize seizures.

But people who followed the keto diet experienced weight loss for some reasons: when you consume carbs, your body retains energy storage fluid (you know if it needs it). But if you're not in the carb department, you lose that water weight. Going overboard on carbohydrates is also easy— but if you load on fat, it can assist reduce cravings as it keeps you satisfied.

That plus the fact that ketosis promotes your body to burn fat, a drastic weight loss can result. "The keto diet started because most people's rules make sense." Nearly all of us want to lose some fat on our body somewhere, and this diet focuses on fat as fuel. "So what foods are keto?

Just because you're not eating all your favorite carb foods, that doesn't mean you're hungry. You will load on healthy fats (like olive oil and avocado), along with plenty of lean protein such as grass-fed beef and chicken, and leafy greens or other non-starchy veggies.

More nice news: snacks are completely permitted (and not just carrot sticks). There's plenty of packaged options for keto fans. FATBAR is among them. They have 200 calories, 16 grams of fat, and four grams of net carbs. They are made of coconut, pea protein, sunflower seeds, cashew butter, cocoa butter, and chia seeds.

For coffee drinkers mourning their vanilla lattes loss, an option is a bulletproof coffee. This is your standard coffee but added with grass-fed butter and medium-chain triglycerides (MCT) oil to help boost healthy A.M fats.

To satisfy your sweet tooth, if you're looking for something, keto fat bombs have a solid following. As the name implies, these are small snacks high in fat and low in carbs, so you can be on-point with your diet even when you indulge.

And if you can't survive without your pasta, there's plenty of products out there, like the organic black bean spaghetti of Explore Cuisine that gives you the pasta experience without the carbs. There are also tons of keto-friendly restaurants— like Red Lobster, Olive Garden, and Texas Roadhouse — that can allow you to have a night out without ketosis.

Chapter 25
Rules For A Headache-
Free Ketogenic Diet

This is MUCH more fat than most individuals eat. Comparison, a normal American diet feels like 50% carbohydrate, 15% protein, and 35% fat.

And the ketogenic diet can be intimidating. You see how much fat you need to consume, and worry about what you consume at your meals and prevent attempting. Or, try all the calories a few days before giving up because it takes too much mental energy.

But it's not tough or frightening. After doing it now for six weeks and monitoring almost everything I've consumed, as well as my ketone concentrations, I've come up with some simple rules that worked to stick to a headache-free ketogenic diet.

Rule 1: No Carbs It's self-explanatory.

No food, except vegetables and avocados, can be regarded carbs. You get that~25 g per day, but that's going to get used to the one or two grams of carbohydrates you eat during the day.

If you have something you eat carbohydrate on top of everything else, it will bring you over your allowance, and you may not get ketosis.

Rule 2: Have a Fatty Breakfast

Where most people fail to get ketosis, they go through their day trying to follow the diet, then reach the evening and realize they don't have enough fat and have to drink heavy cream to make up for it. Yuck.

Instead, load as much of your fat as possible during "breakfast," which implies getting 4 cups of keto coffee as I work out in the morning.

Usually ghee, coffee with butter or black tea, or MCT oil. If you care to mix it up somewhat, I also like mushroom coffee together with any of the fats in it, and if the ordinary oil provides you catastrophe pants, you can try MCT oil powder.

But if you like an ordinary breakfast, it's fairly easy: bacon, eggs, avocado, one or two keto coffees. If you've got 3 eggs, its 15 g fat. 4 Bacon slices about 15 g. Half Avocado 15. Each keto-cup is 14 g.

Your goal is to get at least one-third of your morning fat, so you don't have to worry about it later.

You can calculate your TDEE and then find out what 70% of that is in grams of fat... Or just leave a straightforward rule: your target weight is how many grams of fat you should have.

If you weigh 160lbs and try to reach 150lbs, you should have 150 g of fat all day and shoot at least 50 g for breakfast. If you weigh 110 and attempt to get 100, you should have 100 g of fat all day long, and breakfast at least 33.

Since most of the breakfast foods we've been looking at are within 15 g of fat range, we can make the rule simpler: split your target weight by 30, round up, and that's how many "fat servings" you should have for breakfast.

A fat serving would be:

Eggs - 3 pcs

bacon - 4 slices

avocado - half

1 coffee or tea with a tablespoon of butter / MCT oil / ghee / heavy cream

Once you find out what your number is and discover a dinner combination you never have to think about it again. I'm looking forward to a soft buttery coffee now, and you'll appreciate it too.

Rule 3: Two fatty fist-making fist.

That's how much, twice a day. That's about 1 lb or 16 oz of complete steak, which has precisely how much protein I need to reach my proportions. If you're lower, it's more like 12 oz, about the quantity you need. If you're larger, you'd get 20 or 24 oz.

It's not ideal, but it's an easy start. Instead of constantly attempting to find out the amount of protein you are getting, remember getting two fatty meat fists a day.

The finest meats are:

- Beef (avoiding super lean ground beef)
- Lamb
- Skin-on chicken thigh
- Pork
- Salmon
- Eggs

Rule 4: One fat in each meal

You'll get most of your fat from your fatty breakfast and fatty meats, but you'll still need to add a little more to each meal to make sure you achieve your objective.

It's easiest to add salad dressing, cheese,or nuts. You'll get the fat you need if you can get a couple of cheese, pecans or wlanuts or add 1 to 2 tbsp caesar, olive oil, or ranch dressing to your salad.

Rule 5: Follow and adjust

If you can follow these four guidelines, you should get ketosis and lose fat. But to make sure you do it, it enables monitor some degree. Weight tracking is easiest. If your weight falls, you're likely correct.

Some ketone pee strips are the next simplest way. These will alter colors depending on your ketosis. They're not perfect, but they're going to give you a rough concept of getting into keto.

The third best way is to get my blood ketone testing machine. This lets you see very obviously if you're in ketosis or not, so you understand how well you're on the diet. And what if you don't use one of these exams and diet? Don't you lose weight or keto? Try three things in order: don't consume carbs. No sweeteners, no dressings, no high-carb nuts.

Reduce food intake. You may have too much meat, cut it back to 1/2 fist.

Reduce all-intake. You don't want to reduce the fat ratio, so the last thing to try (mainly if you don't lose weight) is eating less.

Chapter 26
How To Beat Keto Flu

If you do experience insomnia and irritability, your cortisol levels have jumped. Don't worry: as you adjust to using fat and ketones as a new fuel source, your cortisol levels should fall to their old levels.

To beat keto flu, try these remedies.

Hydrate daily. To determine the minimum water required, use your current body weight and divide it by two. It's how many ounces you need. For example, if you weigh 140 pounds, you should target 70 ounces of water a day.

Bone broth adds water to your diet and a dose of electrolytes (sodium and potassium) to offset some of your cellular discomforts. Here's our bone broth recipe.

Electrolyte supplement.

Replenishing your electrolytes is a great way to start feeling faster. Key players are magnesium, : potassium, and sodium. If you don't get enough of them from your diet, which can be hard on low-carb, incorporate them as supplements.

Eat fat, especially MCTs. Higher fat consumption can accelerate your adaptation phase. One caveat: Before reaching the liver, most fats must pass through your lymph system to your heart, muscles and fat cells.

They can only be converted into ketones for body use as source of fuel. MCT oil case is different because after digestion it goes straight to the liver — just like carbs — so it can be used immediately.

Rest well. A sound night's sleep is very good at overcoming keto flu. It ultimately keeps your cortisol levels in check, lowering your flu symptoms. Aim 7-9 hours a night.

Exercise (mildly), meditate. The second word: mild. Yeah, mild. Here, the goal is to reduce cortisol levels, so anything that can relieves stress will surely help. Gentle walks or yoga can be tricky. If exercise is not for you, try meditating. It's probably best not to go full-on in the gym until you adjust to the keto diet.

Activate charcoal. Activated charcoal detoxifies your body as you shed fat. Charcoal binds to chemicals that have positive charges, including many toxic molds, BPA and pesticides.

Exogenous complement ketone. By increasing blood ketone concentrations, exogenous ketones assist fatigue and increase power levels. Note that they are not a replacement for a adequate keto diet, although they may assist you bring it on a knot— especially flu.

If you choose this path, target smaller doses of your supplement to be spread over the first 3 to 5 days of keto flu.

If everything fails, boost your consumption. Increasing fat won't prevent symptoms of keto flu for some. If that's the case — and you've tested your boundaries by adding plenty fat and still experience flu symptoms— you'll just want a bit of your carb consumption.

Chapter 27
Achieve Success With Advanced Ketogenic Diet

The Ketogenic diet entails drastically reducing carbohydrate consumption and simultaneously increasing protein in the amount necessary to keep muscle mass with calorie ratios approximating to 50 %, 30% curative fats and 20 % low glycemic index carbohydrates .

The general dietary guidelines involve avoidance of high carbohydrate foods like potatoes, bread, pasta, rice etc. as well as most of basic carbohydrates like honey, sugar, and fruit juice.

Protein is included in each meal as this will help to reduce appetite, regulate blood sugar levels and maintain lean muscle mass. Examples of protein foods include fish, eggs, chicken, turkey, meat, cheese, tofu and tempeh.

Protein beverages such as whey protein isolate or soy milk might be used. Soy protein is particularly valuable as it has been shown to decrease fat levels, stimulate thyroid hormone production, and promote fat loss, due to the phytoestrogens and essential fatty acids it contains.

Irregular fat intake is also essential since this enhances fat burning from the body while reducing fatty acids synthesis in the body which both enhance fat loss. Optimal resources of fats include fish oil, avocado, flaxseed oil, olive oil, seeds and nuts.

To provide balanced nutrition, minerals, vitamins, and fiber and also to promote detox it is also essential to consume 3-4 cups of low carbohydrate vegetables or salad daily with one optional serve of fruit daily.

When starting a Ketogenic diet program, you may experience some distress such as headaches, fatigue, irritability,and hunger for your initial 2-7 days, nevertheless thereafter it is very simple to stick to this diet and it actually reduces appetite, increases energy levels and carbohydrate cravings.

The Ketogenic diet produces excellent results when followed consistently. Long term success is much more likely possible if a holistic approach is adopted that addresses exercise, daily diet, nutritional supplements and psychological factors in addition to some specific health challenges which are unique to the individual.

When the ideal body fat percentage is attained the diet may be gradually corrected to include more complicated carbohydrates such as starchy vegetables, whole grains, and fruit whilst as much as you can avoiding other simple carbs such as sugar, honey, and refined flours. Simultaneously it's essential to ensure that protein is included in each meal.

This more relaxed form of dietary approach could be kept indefinitely in combination with a regular exercise program to ensure that body composition and weight remain stable.

Though a ketogenic diet has been used to greatly improve people's wellbeing, there are some out there who don't share the majority's way of thinking. However, why is that exactly?

Since we can remember we've been taught that the only way to get rid of this excess weight was to stop eating the fat packed foods which we're accustomed to eating daily.

So instructing people to eat healthy fats, you can surely understand why some people would be skeptical as to why and how you'd eat more fat to attain weight lost and attain it fast. This notion goes against everything we have ever known about weight reduction.

When an average person consume foods full of carbs, their entire body takes those carbohydrates and converts them to glucose as this serves as your body's important source of fuel. Whilst on a Keto diet, all carbs consumed forces your body to use other forms of energy to keep the body functioning properly.

A perfect Keto diet should consist of 5-10% Carbs, 70-80% Fat, 20-25% Protein,. You should not be consuming more than 20g of carbohydrates per day to keep to the normal Ketogenic diet.

Ketogenic diet programs continue to be highly regarded in numerous arenas as highly effective, maintainable weight reduction diet programs. Below are a few suggestions to maximize the success of a ketogenic diet plan.

1.) Drink a lot of water.

While on a ketogenic diet plan, the body has a tough time keeping as a lot of water as it needs, so being effectively hydrated is definitely vital.

A lot of pros suggest that males consumption no less than three liters of drinks daily, even though the figure for females is 2.2 liters daily. A great signal of proper hydration will be the color of the urine. If the urine is light or clear yellow, you are probably properly hydrated. Keep a container of water and you wherever you go!

2.) Do not overlook the fat!

To put it simply, our bodies require fuel to function. Whenever we restrict the carbohydrate intake, particularly to levels which cause ketosis, our bodies require another energy source. Since protein isn't an effective supply of energy, our bodies use fat.

Any fat you consume while in ketosis is utilized for energy, which makes it extremely hard to store body fat while in ketosis. Go for unsaturated and healthy fats as frequently as possible: foods as avocados, nuts, olives, and seeds are perfect.

3.) Find the carb limit.

Dieters will need to adhere to a tight low carbohydrate diet that involves taking under 20 grams of carbs each day. Some other dieters will find that they can comfortably remain in ketosis while consuming fifty, seventy-five, or a hundred grams of carbohydrates.

The sole way to know beyond doubt is error and trial. Any brand or purchase Ketostix of ketone urinalysis strips and also learn the carbohydrate limit. If you discover you have a little bit of wiggle room, it is going to make sticking to the diet a lot easier.

4.) Be sensible about liquor.

Among the fantastic facets of the ketogenic diet plan is the fact that you can drink liquor while on it while not throwing your fat loss far off course.

You can drink unsweetened liquors like brandy, cognac, scotch, whiskey, gin, tequila, rum, and vodka, and the rare low carb beer. Pick low carb mixers and drink a lot of water to remain hydrated, as hangovers are notoriously unhealthy while in ketosis. And don't forget, calories still count, therefore do not get a little obsessive. Most things in small amounts.

5.) Be patient.

Even though the ketogenic diet plan is acknowledged for fast weight reduction, particularly in the first phases of the diet, weight reduction is surely a slow, time-consuming procedure. Do not freak out if the machine does not display weight loss, and shows small industry increases, because of a short time.

Chapter 28
Tips To Make Ketogenic Diet Work

Standard keto: Eat very low carb (less than 50 grams per day), every day. Some adherents consume 20 grams a day.

Consume high-fat, low-carbon (less than 50 grams of net carbs per day) 5-6 days a week. Have carb refeed day 7 (about 150 grams). Bulletproof type of diet falls within this category but tweaks do keto for better results with, protein fasting, intermittent fasting and low-inflammation foods.

You follow the normal keto diet, but before a high-intensity exercise, eat extra carbs 30 minutes to an hour. Glucose is designed to boost effectiveness and return to ketosis after practice. If your keto gym energy suffers, this eating style may work for you.

Dirty keto: This keto type follows an identical ratio of carbs, proteins, fats, just like the regular keto diet, but with a twist even though it does not matter from where it comes. Dinner could be Pepsi's Big Mac bunless diet. Learn about diet and how it works.

Consume high-fat, 100 to 150 grms of net carbs everyday. With this diet, women usually do best— sometimes carbs restriction can tamper with hormonal function. Some athletes discover carbs burning out on exercise days with less than 100 grams.

First, check with your physician before making any significant dietary adjustments.

Try at least one month's keto styles.

Track your carbs, fat and protein using MyFitnessPal and My Macros+.

Set fat-and-carbon objectives instead of worrying about calories. Eat up, listen to your body.

Are you on a weekly carb refeed, or are you better on a complete ketogenic diet?

Burn when you dip below 100 grams a day? Low-carb differences exist, and some individuals feel their best with distinct eating styles. Find a nice equilibrium for your biology.

Generally speaking, a ketogenic diet is completely secure for many people— but there are a few side effects to watch out for: Carbs need dehydration and muscle cramps. Not fat. You do not store much water on a keto diet, and instead of keeping it, your kidneys do actively expel sodium. This implies

Dehydrated eating keto is simple, particularly in the first weeks. Dehydration and low electrolytes can also begin cramping.

Double on magnesium, sodium and potassium, your body's three primary electrolytes, and make sure you drink additional water. Particularly important when operating on keto. Staying hydrated also helps prevent symptoms of keto flu.

Many individuals report struggling to process carbs when they consume a rigorous long-term, meaningful keto diet. If you rarely eat carbs, your insulin pathways don't have to run. It's like maintaining daylight on— a waste of electricity.

Your body seems to de-regulate insulin (the hormone telling your cells to use carbs for fuel) after a while of strict keto. Some components of your body flourish on glucose, such as glial cells that handle repair and immune function. If you have great fat cells and terrible carbs, you won't operate at complete strength.

Do this: try carb cycling by eating 150 grams of quality carbs one day a week.

Insomnia Keto and sleep problems are not researched, but some individuals report keto waking up midnight. If you find that you have trouble sleeping on keto (and bulletproof sleep hacks don't assist), you may be better off eating some high-quality carbs.

Strictly speaking, these problems are prevalent and are a significant component of why the Bulletproof Diet contains some quality carbs.

Insomnia is a dietary side effect: bring 1 teaspoon of raw honey before bed.

If you consume less than 20 grams of carbs a day, getting enough fiber can be difficult. Low fiber consumption can cause constipation, irritable bowel syndrome (IBS), and enhanced risk of colon cancer.

Keto diet needs additional fiber to remain regular, such as leafy greens: make sure most of your keto diet carbs come from leafy, colourful, fiber-rich plants.

Eat more fiber-rich foods like sweet potatoes, butternut squash with a cyclical keto diet.

Try a prebiotic fiber like InnerFuel, which feeds useful gut bacteria.

Make sure you get 2-2 1/2 teaspoons of salt a day to keep enough water to keep your bowels regular.

Load potassium and magnesium and Stay hydrated— vital electrolytes can be found in avocado, spinach,and supplements.

Keep nutritional. Track what you eat, see what you do, and don't digest well.

Exercise can assist remain regular, supporting the digestive tract.

Diarrhea

Some individuals experience keto-diarrhea on the reverse end of the spectrum, particularly if they're not used to a higher-fat diet.

Do this: begin slowly with MCT oils: This oil is a saturated fatty acid that that gives your body rapid ketone energy. It helps increase your body as it adapts. Your digestive system may take some time to use MCT oils. Start 1 tsp and operate from there.

Add digestive enzyme: do not digest fats correctly. Try lipase, an enzyme that digests body fat, or hydrochloric acid (HCL), which helps increase stomach acid and digestion.

Keto rash

Itchy rash on the neck, chest, back, or armpit area can lead in very small numbers of people attempting keto. Keto rash, referred to as Prurigo pigmentosa, is not life-threatening. Exact causes are not yet recognized, but as prospective triggers, scientists point to variations in hormones, gut bacteria or allergens.

Keto Rash Do this: check with your doctor and try these tips to deal with keto rash:

Bring back carbs: you do not require a bread binge, whether a sudden change to a keto way of life is brought by a rash, you can reintroduce some high-quality healthy, carbs such as pumpkin, yams, carrots, sweet potatoes, and butternut squash.

Like all rashes, it can worsen with sweat, friction,or heat. Do not worsen irritated skin by putting on breathable garments , loose-fitting garments, and avoiding scented products, perfumes, or sweat-inducing workout until the skin can cure.

Support your skin: Anti-inflammatory foods and supplements can help increase your healing time and calm your rash. Try to include products like this turmeric latte, DHA omega-3 supplement, or these top 5 healthy skin nutrients.

Changing from burning sugar to fat is a natural response your body undergoes. Keto flu generally hits the 24 to 48 hours mark. Symptoms comprises of headache, fog, muscle soreness, insomnia, bad concentrate, irritability, sugar cravings.

Keto flu do affects more people than others. Before going to keto, eating low in starch and refined sugar, you may experience mild symptoms only. An elevated sugar and carbohydrate diet may produce higher withdrawal symptoms (particularly sugar).

Conclusion

Ketogenic's is a high-fat diet that encourages your body to burn fat stores. Yes, you heard that right, a high-fat diet that burns your existing fat. Sounds like a pretty good deal, but before you run to the local Krispy Kreme and start scarfing down crullers in the name of ketogenic's, let's get some background information first.

The ketogenic diet developed in the 1920s as a potential epilepsy therapy. The diet replaces carbohydrates with fat because carbohydrates break down into glucose, which can trigger epileptic seizures, while fat breaks down into fatty acids and ketone bodies, which are then used to replace energy in the brain.

The diet lost its popularity with daytime anticonvulsant drugs. In the 1990s, the son of Jim Abrahams, a Hollywood producer, found relief for his epilepsy through this innovative dietary approach. Now, more and more people choose ketogenic diets for their own weight-loss goals.

Everyone is looking to turn the clock back. To get that figure they had in high school. Who thought the answer lies in high-fat foods? It seems, however, that may be the case. Once the body begins to use fat as a source of energy rather than carbohydrates, your body has entered ketosis. In this state, you feel less hungry.

The body using the fat as energy combined with your reduced appetite can result in the dieter's rapid and significant weight loss. So, we're talking about replacing carbohydrates with fat, but what exactly will qualify for this type of enhanced diet?

The list is long and includes bacon, butter, mayonnaise, hot dogs, cream, nuts and more. While eating fatty foods, you try to stay away from any of the carb-loaded foods. They include almost anything made with sugar; cake, pastry, cookies, candy and white flour foods, including pasta and white bread.

The diet sounds simple enough, but remember, this diet was developed by doctors to treat patients with epilepsy. A doctor generally monitored it, and it is recommended that you heed similar advice. Looking for a better body and fat loss, many of us will try anything.

A ketogenic diet may help you achieve your goals, but it can be risky. High blood pressure, high cholesterol, and other medical conditions may occur during such a diet.

Combining the diet with a rigorous and consistent exercise routine will certainly help limit, but not completely avoid, the existence and severity of such conditions.